100 Questions s About Kid and Hypertension

Raymond R. Townsend, MD

Director of the Research Hypertension Program
Hospital of the University of Pennsylvania
Renal Division

Debbie L. Cohen, MD

Director of the Clinical Hypertension Program
Hospital of the University of Pennsylvania
Renal Division
Assistant Professor of Medicine
University of Pennsylvania

JONES AND BARTLETT PUBLISHERS
Sudbury, Massachusetts
BOSTON   TORONTO   LONDON   SINGAPORE

World Headquarters
Jones and Bartlett Publishers
40 Tall Pine Drive
Sudbury, MA 01776
978-443-5000
info@jbpub.com
www.jbpub.com

Jones and Bartlett Publishers
Canada
6339 Ormindale Way
Mississauga, Ontario L5V 1J2
CANADA

Jones and Bartlett Publishers
International
Barb House, Barb Mews
London W6 7PA
UK

Jones and Bartlett's books and products are available through most bookstores and online booksellers. To contact Jones and Bartlett Publishers directly, call 800-832-0034, fax 978-443-8000, or visit our website, www.jbpub.com.

Substantial discounts on bulk quantities of Jones and Bartlett's publications are available to corporations, professional associations, and other qualified organizations. For details and specific discount information, contact the special sales department at Jones and Bartlett via the above contact information or send an email to specialsales@jbpub.com.

The authors, editor, and publisher have made every effort to provide accurate information. However, they are not responsible for errors, omissions, or for any outcomes related to the use of the contents of this book and take no responsibility for the use of the products and procedures described. Treatments and side effects described in this book may not be applicable to all people; likewise, some people may require a dose or experience a side effect that is not described herein. Drugs and medical devices are discussed that may have limited availability controlled by the Food and Drug Administration (FDA) for use only in a research study or clinical trial. Research, clinical practice, and government regulations often change the accepted standard in this field. When consideration is being given to use of any drug in the clinical setting, the health care provider or reader is responsible for determining FDA status of the drug, reading the package insert, and reviewing prescribing information for the most up-to-date recommendations on dose, precautions, and contraindications, and determining the appropriate usage for the product. This is especially important in the case of drugs that are new or seldom used.

Production Credits
Executive Publisher: Christopher Davis
Production Director: Amy Rose
Associate Editor: Kathy Richardson
Editorial Assistant: Jessica Acox
Associate Production Editor: Leah Corrigan
V.P. of Manufacturing and
   Inventory Control: Therese Connell

Associate Marketing Manager: Ilana Goddess
Composition: Lynn L'Heureux
Cover Design: Kate Ternullo
Cover Images: © Yuri Arcurs/ShutterStock, Inc.
   © Rob Marmion/ShutterStock, Inc.
   © GeoM/ShutterStock, Inc.
Printing and Binding: Malloy, Inc.
Cover Printing: Malloy, Inc.

Library of Congress Cataloging-in-Publication Data
Townsend, Raymond R.
  100 questions and answers about kidney disease and hypertension / Raymond Townsend and Debbie L. Cohen -- 1st ed.
    p. cm.
  Includes index.
  ISBN 978-0-7637-5776-2 (alk. paper)
  1. Renal hypertension--Miscellanea. 2. Kidneys--Diseases--Miscellanea. 3. Hypertension--Miscellanea. I. Cohen, Debbie L. II. Title. III. Title: One hundred questions and answers about kidney disease and hypertension.
  RC918.R38T69 2008
  616.1'32--dc22

6048   2008022726

Printed in the United States of America
12 11 10 09 08   10 9 8 7 6 5 4 3 2 1

I would like to dedicate this work to my mentor, Dr. Bob Narins (previously Czar of Education for the American Society of Nephrology and my kidney mentor at Temple University 1982–1984), and Christine Bastl (my research in kidney disease mentor 1983–1984) both of whom set me on the course working in the area of Kidney Disease. I am also indebted to Dr. Edmond Burke (last sighted standing near a car with a flat tire in Brooklyn, NY) whose Irish accent and compelling logic persuaded me to enter the field of kidney disease during my medical residency in the late 1970s. I am extremely grateful to the patients who have taught me so much about kidney disease by sharing their experiences with me over these many years. And last, but most importantly, to my wife of 30 years, Arlene. She has struggled, laughed, and cried with me throughout this adventure we call "marriage" and continues to be my best friend ever.

—Raymond Townsend, MD

I would like to dedicate this book to my alma mater, the University of the Witwatersrand Medical School.

I am eternally grateful for the amazing training I received, particularly the clinical skills that set the foundation for my successful career in the United States. I still hold many of my professors and lecturers in awe. I thank them for imparting their wisdom and serving as role models on how to be a real doctor.

Dr. Townsend and I have worked together for 10 years. He has been an amazing mentor and has constantly urged me to continue to strive for more. He is the smartest person I know. I also dedicate this to my husband, Steven, and our four wonderful sons Joshua, David, Jacob, and Noah, who have lived this journey.

—Debbie Cohen, MD

CONTENTS

Questions 1–8 cover basic information on the kidneys and their function, including:
- What exactly do my kidneys do?
- Where are my kidneys located?
- Is the amount of urine I pass related to my kidney function?

Questions 9–22 are concerned with the signs and symptoms of kidney disease and how it is detected:
- My doctor said I have tiny proteins in my urine. What's that about?
- How is my kidney function measured? When should I see a kidney doctor if I have been told that I have kidney disease?
- When should a patient with abnormal kidney function see a kidney specialist? Can my primary care physician take care of this problem?

Questions 23–33 answer queries related to the connection of high blood pressure and kidney function, such as:
- How common is high blood pressure (hypertension) in people with kidney disease?
- My doctor was concerned that my kidney arteries are blocked. Why would she think that?
- My blood pressure has been very difficult to control. If my blood pressure remains high, will this affect my kidney function?

Chronic kidney disease is very common and currently affects approximately 20 million adults in the United States. This book explains the many complex facets of kidney disease and the management of the various conditions. The authors have a combined 35 years of clinical experience in caring for patients with various types of kidney disease.

PART ONE

General Information About Kidneys

What exactly do my kidneys do?

Where are my kidneys located?

Is kidney disease inherited?

More . . .

1. What exactly do my kidneys do?

That seems like a great question with which to start this book!

Your kidneys have three functions. The first is dealing with all of the fluid that each of us guzzles in the course of the day. Whether you realize it or not, most of us drink between 1 and 2 quarts of fluid a day, not to mention the amount of water that is in our food. Doing some simple math, considering each quart of fluid weighs about 2 pounds, if our kidneys did not excrete that intake daily, we would gain about 4 pounds a day. Think of what would happen in a month. Even the most compulsive devotee of the Jenny Craig diet couldn't hope to battle that kind of weight gain. The first thing kidneys do is make urine, which protects us from massive sogginess on a daily basis.

Uremia

Describes the illness accompanying kidney failure. In kidney failure, urea and other waste products, which are normally excreted into the urine, are retained in the blood.

Hormones

Chemicals made by glands, like the adrenal glands or the pancreas, that signal other tissues to function in a particular manner.

Erythropoietin

A glycoprotein secreted by the kidneys that stimulates the production of red blood cells.

The second function of the kidneys is to filter and get rid of the daily waste product load. It would be inaccurate to say that the kidneys get rid of all the waste products in the course of the day, since that would minimize the role of the liver which handles some of this burden. However, it is fair to say that the kidneys get rid of at least 90 percent of the waste from the body's metabolism, and from the food that we eat each day. When the kidneys fail to get rid of the waste products, we say that a person is developing **uremia**. This word simply means "*ur*ine in the blood (blood is referred to as hema, and the medical suffix becomes '(h)emia')."

Finally, and least likely to be guessed correctly in Trivial Pursuit, the kidneys perform an endocrine function. By that, we mean that they secrete **hormones**. There are at least two very important ones. You'll hear more about them later in this book, but peeking ahead their names are **erythropoietin** (what a mouthful!) and active vitamin D.

Of course, there are a few other things that the kidneys do. These are subsets of the above functions. Perhaps the most noteworthy of which is that the kidneys help control the blood pressure through their ability to get eliminate our daily sodium intake.

Our bloodstream has a delicate balance of about a half dozen or so important minerals, and the kidney adjusts their individual balances flawlessly most of the time.

The kidneys do this through the ability to either excrete the extra water that would otherwise dilute these minerals or conserve the water when we go for long periods without drinking. They also have the good sense to get rid of the minerals we absorb in our diet but do not need.

2. I was born with a single kidney. Does that mean I will have problems later?

Maybe. If you do, it is usually not until you're at least 40 years old, and that's assuming that you were really born with one kidney. Some people are born with two, but an accident or disease may destroy one kidney so that a person functionally has only one remaining kidney. Then, there's that issue of giving one of your kidneys to your parents, your children, your neighbor, the nice man who cuts the lawn, et cetera.

Kidney donation is, in our estimation, one of the most amazing things a person can do for another person. If we didn't think it was safe to take a kidney out, we wouldn't do so many living kidney donations each year. Statistically, the most frequent consequences when a kidney is removed or you're only born with one are that a tiny amount of protein will appear in the urine (see questions 10 and 11) and your blood pressure will usually be a little higher than someone else your age, gender, and approximate weight. At the time we write this, our health-care system at the University of Pennsylvania does between 180 and 200 kidney transplants each year. About 40 percent of these are from people who donate their kidneys, usually to a family member or a spouse. By and large, people do quite well after kidney donation and it's usually not the case that severe amounts of protein in the urine or serious hypertension occurs as a result.

Our bloodstream has a delicate balance of about a half dozen or so important minerals, and the kidney adjusts their individual balances flawlessly most of the time.

Kidney donation is, in our estimation, one of the most amazing things a person can do for another person.

When you think about it, the fact that most people with a single kidney do just fine is a testimony as to how robust these guys we call the kidneys really are.

3. Where are my kidneys located?

Your kidneys are tucked way up under your ribs very near to the back surface of you. When you take a deep breath, the kidneys slide as much as 1 to 2 inches below the ribs. They spend most of their time enjoying the protection your rib cage gives them from daily traumas such as riding the subway, as one of the authors does. The kidneys are pretty soft, and incredibly important, so their location within a bony surrounding makes perfect sense. In relatively thin people, the kidneys are about 1 to 2 inches below the surface of the skin. In a person who has the body type of your typical linebacker on a major league football team, the kidneys are more like 4 or 5 inches below the surface. Figure 1 gives you an idea of their approximate location.

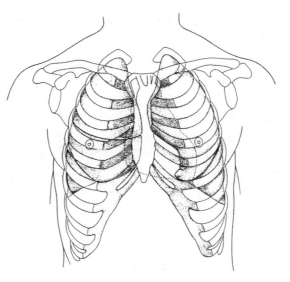

Figure 1. Location of the kidneys in relation to the heart and lungs.

From *100 Questions and Answers About Heart Attack and Related Cardiac Problems*, Edward K Chung, MD, FACP, FACC, Jones and Bartlett Publishers, LLC © 2004.

4. If I have back pain could that come from my kidneys?

Our dollars to your doughnuts says that it's usually not. We say this for two reasons.

First, the kidneys don't have much of a nervous system that detects pain. It isn't like the nerves in your thumb that you don't think about until you miss a nail and hit your thumb with a hammer! That's not to say that the kidneys don't register pain, but they usually do so when they are blocked in some way such as happens with a kidney stone and the little tube connecting them to the bladder (the **ureter**) is dilated or stretched.

Second, muscles and bones just hurt more often. They are what you abuse when you bend over and pick up heavy things the wrong way, or fall asleep in some unnatural position in your reclining chair. From a practical standpoint, it's a whole lot easier to stretch, wrench or twist muscle and bone.

When the kidneys are the source of pain, it has a characteristic we call "colic." This is not the kind of colic a baby has. You have to experience colic yourself in order to appreciate the peculiar characteristics of that kind of pain. Doctors tend to think that when a man experiences colic, it's the closest thing to the pain of labor and delivery that he will ever feel. We will have lots more to say on the topic in Part 7.

Ureter

The ureters are the ducts that carry urine from the kidneys to the urinary bladder, passing anterior to the psoas major. The ureters are muscular tubes that can propel urine along, in the adult, the ureters are usually 25–30 cm long.

5. How big are a person's kidneys?

Interestingly enough, your kidneys are about the size of your hand. Reach your arms straight out like you're stopping traffic, and then tip your hands upwards. From your wrist to your fingertip is about five to six inches in most people. This is the size of normal kidneys in the adult. The kidneys tend to be a little bit thicker than your hands, usually about an inch and a half in thickness and about 3 inches wide.

Ultrasound

Renal ultrasound is a special X-ray of the kidneys, which does not involve exposure to radiation.

Polycystic kidney disease (PKD)

A progressive, genetic disorder of the kidneys. It is characterized by the presence of multiple cysts (hence, "polycystic") in both kidneys.

The most common cause of kidney disease in the United States is diabetes mellitus due to the epidemic of obesity.

Doctors usually measure kidney sizes with an **ultrasound**. When disease strikes the kidneys, it almost always diminishes their size. The exception is when a patient has AIDS. In that situation, the kidneys are usually bigger than normal, and usually with lots of protein in the urine. The other time the kidneys tend to grow in size even though they may be failing in their function is with the adult **polycystic kidney disease** or APKD for short. We will have more to say about that one in Question 50.

6. Is kidney disease inherited?

Sometimes, and sometimes not. The most common cause of kidney disease in the United States is diabetes mellitus due to the epidemic of obesity. We're still not quite sure exactly how much of diabetes, or the tendency toward diabetes is inherited. However, there are several very clear familial syndromes that affect the kidneys. APKD is one of the most common of the inherited forms of kidney disease. APKD accounts for about 1 in 20 patients on dialysis in the United States (roughly 5 percent). With other inherited kidney disease, there are sometimes additional problems besides those directly affecting the kidneys. For example Alport's syndrome has deafness and some problems with the eyes as part of its presentation.

When a disease is inherited, we say it's either dominant or recessive. If it's dominant, then the gene that causes the problem is so potent and important that every child of someone who has APKD has a 50:50 chance of inheriting APKD. In a recessive disorder, you have to get a disease gene from each parent in order to develop the disease.

Geneticists would be shuddering over our simplistic explanation, so we'll finish this question with a disclaimer. The dominant and recessive forms of inherited diseases are useful genetic concepts, but of course there are exceptions. In Question 100, we will talk about this more.

7. Is the amount of urine I pass related to my kidney function?

Nope. Well, there goes a perfectly good old wives' tale. You might need a pencil and paper to follow the logic for our answer. So here goes . . .

Your kidneys receive about one half quart of fluid pumped to them by the heart each minute. They filter about 20 percent of that, or roughly four ounces each minute. Next, they recover about 98 to 99 percent of those four ounces. When you multiply four ounces per minute by 1,440 minutes in a day, you come up with 5,760 ounces every day. The average gallon has 128 ounces, so if your kidneys just filtered and did not recover the filtered fluid, well—you'd be spending an awful lot of time in the bathroom until you disappeared into your own stream! It works out to be about 45 or more gallons per day. Even if your kidneys were only working at five percent, they could still filter several gallons a day and from this they could still generate quite a bit of urine. Many dialysis patients make one to two quarts of urine per day despite the fact that they have almost no measurable kidney function.

On the other hand, when a person makes no urine, that's bad. It's usually not the case that you can have good kidney function and make no urine. This is something of a trick question. When you make no urine, you usually do have some kind of kidney problem. When you pass urine volumes that seem normal, it's no guarantee that everything is hunky-dory when it comes to your kidneys and their ability to filter the blood at what we consider a normal level.

8. Do I need to drink 8 glasses of water per day to maintain good kidney function?

We sincerely hope our spouses do not buy this book. Here goes another old wives' tale. No.

In a deep recess of your skull there resides a tiny little gland called the pituitary. Among the many things that the pituitary gland does is respond when you need fluid. We call this response "thirst." The actual sensation of thirst is registered in another part of the brain. It's up to the pituitary to make appropriate responses when the body needs to get rid of waste products. If you've been playing tennis with that guy you couldn't beat in high school and have gotten dehydrated, your pituitary will bail you out by making a hormone that will help concentrate urine until you come to your senses and (to quote an advertising campaign) "obey your thirst."

Obviously, there is a huge mystique about the eight glasses of water a day. Is it ever indicated? Well, yes, there are a few times when it is a good idea. These are occasions when it's really important to have a dilute urine. One particular instance is when your kidneys form kidney stones. In that circumstance, keeping the urine dilute as possible is a hedge against forming another stone and one of the most important things you can do to prevent future kidney stone occurrence.

Diabetes insipidus

A rare disease resulting from a deficiency of vasopressin (the pituitary hormone that regulates the kidneys) or inability of receptors in the kidney to utilize vasopressin.

While we're dealing with exceptions to the rule, if you don't happen to have that pituitary hormone (whose name is antidiuretic hormone or ADH for short) then it's a good idea to carry around as much water as you physically can, since you will need it. We call that disorder **diabetes insipidus**. Fortunately, there are multiple ways to replace ADH, consequently folks afflicted with this disorder no longer need to purchase huge amounts of stock in Evian® or some other water supplier.

PART TWO

Diagnosis of Kidney Disease

What does blood in the urine mean?

How is my kidney function measured? When should I see a kidney doctor if I have been told that I have kidney disease?

If I still pass a lot of urine does this mean my kidney function is still good?

More . . .

9. What does blood in the urine mean?

Well, it's usually not good news. Its meaning can vary from trivial to really important. In the case of a relatively young woman, it could be a contaminant from her monthly menstrual period. For a guy, blood in the urine tends to be a bit more ominous. In Table 1, we cite the most common causes of blood in the urine.

Table 1: Common causes of blood in the urine (hematuria)

Disorder that can cause hematuria	Common age range affected
*Urinary tract infection	Any age
*Kidney stones	20 and older
Exercise	15 to 50
Trauma	15 and older
Glomerular diseases	Any age
*Prostate enlargement	Men: 40 and older
Polycystic kidney disease (adult)	20 and older
Sickle cell trait or disease	10 and older
*Cancer of kidney, ureters, bladder	40 and older
*Unexplained (no cause found)	0 and older

The more common causes are marked with an *.

Hematuria

Blood in the urine.

When blood does make its way into the urine, it may be in amounts too small to be visible to the naked eye. We call this "microscopic **hematuria**," where the word microscopic means we can only see it when we look at the urine under the microscope. In some cases, the amount of bleeding is visible to the point of making the urine red in color. If this ever happens to you, don't panic—at least not at first. One drop of blood will be readily evident in a bucket (or toilet bowl) of urine. It often looks worse than it is, at least from the amount of blood a person is losing.

By and large, visible amounts of bleeding in the urine are typically seen with kidney stones, tumors, and conditions like sickle cell disease. Microscopic amounts of blood in the urine may be due to intrinsic kidney diseases, there are a lot of them—many questions in this book will deal with disorders that have microscopic hematuria as part of their presentation. Sometimes, microscopic hematuria will have no diagnosis associated with it and may be present for years. Both of the authors follow several patients where they've never really gotten to the bottom of where the blood is coming from despite fairly exhaustive evaluations.

Hematuria, or blood in the urine, is not a normal finding. Its importance can range from fairly innocuous to much worse. There are lots of things that can be done to pursue the cause. The simplest things are medical history and the physical examination. These usually don't hurt, and can yield a diagnosis much of the time. We reserve the scary sounding stuff (like "kidney biopsies") for the most difficult cases where we are stumped as to what the cause is, or when it's important to know a specific thing like the exact kind of kidney disease present because that will be important for how it's treated. There is a lot more to say on this topic and we'll talk more about it in future questions.

Hematuria, or blood in the urine, is not a normal finding. Its importance can range from fairly innocuous to much worse.

10. I was told I have protein in the urine. I was also told my kidney function was normal. What does that mean?

There are basically three ways that the kidneys can seem to be abnormal. We'll have more to say about this later in Question 15, so here is the executive version. Your kidneys can look funny when imaged by an ultrasound or an X-ray. Your kidneys may have reduced function as measured by blood tests that specifically give that kind of information. They may show abnormalities in the urine such as blood or protein (which are usually not detectable) and yet look normal when imaged and appear fine when their function is tested.

Having protein in the urine can occur because of a change in the filtering units that normally restrict the loss of protein. Of course nothing is perfect, so a little protein does get past even the staunchest filters. The reserve corps is the next segment in **nephrons**, and we have a lot to say about those guys later in Question 19. Take a peak at Figure 3 in Question 19 and don't worry about the terminology just yet. The next segment is the tubule, which is where the little bit of protein that gets through the filters is corralled and returned to the body. It's possible for the filters to leak a little more than usual, yet filter and eliminate the waste products just fine so the kidney function appears okay. To the degree that the tubules pick up the slack, nothing out of the ordinary appears in the urine. Sooner or later, the amount of protein leaking through the filters can overwhelm their hearty defensive linemen and protein starts to show up when the urine is checked. You don't lose kidney function until either the number of filters is significantly reduced or until the tubules get so damaged from trying to salvage all the protein that they shut down. That often takes years to happen, and our goal is to try and minimize the proteinuria when we find it so that the filters and the tubules continue to excrete the daily waste product load for many years to come.

Oh, and yes, you do. That is, you do have kidney disease if the protein loss lasts more than three months. Question 19 will reveal all.

11. My doctor said I have tiny proteins in my urine. What's that about?

What your doctor meant was **microalbuminuria**. This refers to the amount, not the size, of **albumin** in the urine. Albumin is the same protein as that found in the white of an egg. It's one of the most important proteins in the body, and your kidneys work pretty hard to keep you from losing any in the urine. Nonetheless, a tiny bit escapes from everybody, usually in the range of less than 10 mg per day. If you think that a

Nephrons

The nephron is the functional unit of the kidney, responsible for the actual purification and filtration of the blood.

Microalbuminuria

A type of albuminaria that is characterized by relatively low levels of albumin in the urine (between 30 and 300 mg in 1 day).

Albumin

Component of protein in the blood, low levels of serum albumin reflect poor nutritional status.

normal aspirin is 365 mg, you can see the 10 mg of albumin is very small.

When your doctor or a laboratory technician checks your urine for protein, they use a **dipstick**. The dipstick test only detects amounts of albumin that are much higher than the amount we're talking about in this question. To have your urine show albumin on a dipstick, you need at least 30 mg per deciliter of urine, or at least 300 mg in a day. If you lose 10 mg in the course of the day in 1 or 2 quarts of urine, the actual concentration of albumin is more like 1 mg per deciliter. A quart has about 10 deciliters so you can see that it's pretty amazing we are able to detect such little amounts of this important protein. We think when you lose more than 30 mg of albumin in the urine in the course of the day that that moves you from the "clearly normal" group into the "maybe something is going on" group.

When people have serious kidney conditions such as diabetic kidney disease, they frequently have lots of proteinuria (protein present in their urine). In the last 20 years, we have learned that even these small amounts of albumin, well below the dipstick radar range but still above the normal range, tell us something about a person's health status. They reflect **endothelial function**. What this means is that the blood vessels aren't behaving quite normally, and a little extra albumin is leaking out into the urine. People who have microalbuminuria are at higher risk for cardiovascular diseases, like heart attack. It's that the blood vessels are showing signs of modest but important damage.

A couple of words of caution about microalbuminuria. First, if you have a meal of Chinese food with a liberal dose of soy sauce, you can push up the urine albumin losses. For reasons that aren't totally clear, high salt intakes increases albumin excretion in the urine. So does exercise, fever, and urinary tract infections. Moreover, because you have microalbuminuria on one occasion doesn't guarantee it will happen again, so we

---

Dipstick

A chemically sensitive strip of paper used to identify one or more constituents (such as glucose or protein) of urine by immersion into a urine specimen.

When people have serious kidney conditions such as diabetic kidney disease, they frequently have lots of proteinuria (protein present in their urine).

Endothelial function

Functional ability of the lining of blood vessels.

usually do a second sample to make sure it's really present, and sometimes three samples are necessary. Fortunately, there are medications that seem to undo the processes that lead to microalbuminuria and reduce the urine excretion of albumin back to normal in many cases. We'll have more to say on that later—so please stick around!

David's comments:

I had questions when I first recognized my urine was looking different. I noticed all these little bubbles when I was urinating. Fortunately, I acted and made an appointment to see a renal specialist. Dr Cohen put me through some routine testing and it was determined I had proteinuria. An abnormal amount of protein was spilling into my urine instead of being absorbed into my bloodstream. Dr Cohen treated the condition with the proper medications. Within a week, my proteinuria count started coming down. The decrease was dramatic. Over time, high proteinuria counts can cause damage to the kidneys.

12. My doctor said my creatinine is a little high. What is creatinine?

Creatinine is a waste product that is made mostly by muscle. It comes from a compound called creatine which you might have noticed in a General Nutrition Center or other health food store. Creatine is used in energy **metabolism** in many tissues. Muscle, as you know, is very active and, consequently, uses a lot of energy so it has loads of creatine from which creatinine is ultimately generated. Once creatinine is made, it's a metabolic dead end and it's the kidney's job to get rid of it. It's made in pretty steady fashion so it's excreted in pretty steady fashion. The blood level of creatinine is simply the balance between the amount you make and the amount that passes through your kidneys into the urine. When you begin to lose kidney function then the creatinine level starts to increase.

Metabolism

The minimal energy expended to maintain respiration, circulation, peristalsis, muscle tonus, body temperature, glandular activity, and the other vegetative functions of the body.

From a dietary standpoint, one of the principal sources of creatinine intake is hamburger. When you think about it, most meat is muscle. It makes a lot of sense that there would be some creatinine in meat products. However, these are a relatively small contribution when compared to the large amount of muscle mass we have so we tend to ignore creatinine intake from the diet when using the serum creatinine concentration to evaluate kidney function in patients.

David's comments:

I have come to learn the creatinine level is really my scorecard. The creatinine level tracks how efficiently my kidneys are ridding my body of toxins and waste. And the wait for the call from the doctor's office to inform me of the new creatinine count is always a source of angst and concern. Getting a good number is better than my mother's meatballs (well almost as good anyway).

13. My doctor said he found blood in my urine. Should I see a kidney specialist? Should I see a urologist?

Blood is found in the urine in one of two circumstances.

In one situation, the urine is actually tinged pink or even red. The discovery is followed by a panicked phone call from the patient to the doctor (or the doctor's answering service) who recommends that the patient either come into the office or the emergency room. We call this gross **hematuria**, not because it's "gross" as such terminology might be used by a teenager, but because it's simply, or grossly, evident.

The other situation is more in line with the nature of this question. In this circumstance, blood in the urine is found not because the urine has any particular color change but because a test was done. This test found a very small amount, or microscopic, amount of blood in the urine. This kind of urinary blood loss is **occult**. It would not have been evident without the test. The testing is done in two steps. In the first

Occult

Not manifest or detectable by clinical methods alone and also not present in macroscopic amounts

Hemoglobin

Iron-containing protein present in the blood that is present in red blood cells and gives the cells the red color. It is a transporter of oxygen in the blood.

Centrifuge

A piece of equiptment, driven by a motor, that puts an object in rotation around a fixed axis.

Myoglobin

The oxygen-transporting protein of muscle, resembling blood hemoglobin in function but with only one heme as part of the myoglobin.

Prescription

An instruction from a licensed clinician like a physician, an advanced practice nurse, a midwife, or a physician's assistant that provides for a medication or device to be issued by a pharmacy.

step, a plastic strip with a bunch of little square cotton pads on it is dipped into the urine. Hence the incredibly clever name: a dipstick. One of these small cotton squares contains orthotoluidine blue, which responds to the presence of **hemoglobin** by turning green. Hemoglobin is that part of the red blood cell which gives it the red color because of the iron atom in the center of each hemoglobin molecule. We usually confirm the finding on the dipstick by looking at the urine after we have placed it in the **centrifuge** which forces all the formed elements in the urine, like blood cells, to the bottom of the test tube into which we had poured the urine. After this centrifugation, we pour off the upper part and then take a careful look at all the stuff in the bottom of the tube. At this point, we place this cloudy little droplet on a microscope slide and look at it. With the help of the powerful magnification of the microscope, we can then determine that the color change on the dipstick was really do to the presence of red blood cells. Once in a while it is not. In that situation hemoglobin's cousin **myoglobin** is the cause. It looks like hemoglobin but it comes from muscle, not red blood cells.

Once it's determined that blood is present in the urine whether microscopic or gross we tend to pursue its cause.

14. How is my kidney function measured? When should I see a kidney doctor if I have been told that I have kidney disease?

Believe it or not, this is a somewhat difficult question to answer. The simple response is that we measure serum creatinine, check to see if the result falls in the normal range, and if the result falls outside of the normal range, we say you have a problem. Let us illustrate with an example.

Let's take a hypothetical patient. She's a 46-year-old, African-American woman with high blood pressure, for which she takes medicine. She sees her new doctor for the first time and that doctor sends her to the hospital lab with a **prescription** for a serum creatinine concentration blood test. She comes back to her doctor in 2 weeks to have her blood pressure checked and to hear the results of her blood test. It turns out that her creatinine is reported by the lab to be one point one milligram per deciliter (1.1 mg/dL). What it means is that every deciliter (that's about 1/10 of a quart) of her blood has 1.1 mg of creatinine (see Question 12 for more on creatinine). When you look at the lab report it says that the normal range for creatinine is 0.5 to 1.5 mg/dl. We would think that her kidney function would be normal since her value fell right smack dab in the middle of the normal range. However, although creatinine is pretty good as a marker of kidney function we also know that changes occur in how creatinine is made and excreted as we get older. In recent years, we have tried to factor in things like age and the fact that women tend to have a smaller muscle mass (and thus make less creatinine on a day to day basis) compared to men. Moreover, people of African-American ancestry tend to have different muscle mass than those of Caucasian ancestry. A group of very smart doctors got together and measured kidney function with a very tedious test called a GFR. **GFR** is medspeak for glomerular filtration rate. We bet that's clear as mud right now. When you ask a doctor how to define what kidney function is, the doctor will say kidney function is related to the glomerular filtration rate or GFR. Since we think that a primary job description of the kidney is to filter the blood and generate urine, we say that it's function depends on how much blood the kidney actually filters, thus, the "F" in GFR. This very smart group of doctors measured the GFR with a radioactive tracer called **iothalamate**. This radioactive tracer was given in very tiny amounts, with less radiation exposure to the patient then they might have experienced by having a CT scan. The only way iothalamate leaves the body is through filtration by the kidney. The filter units in the kidney are called **glomeruli**. We see your mind connecting the dots here with the word glomeruli and the G in GFR. Strong work! So, completing this analogy, the *rate* at which the iothalamate is filtered by the glomeruli and excreted becomes the R in GFR. Once the GFR is known, then the trick was to figure out exactly how to relate

When you ask a doctor how to define what kidney function is, the doctor will say kidney function is related to the glomerular filtration rate or GFR.

GFR

Determines level of kidney function and stage of kidney disease.

Iothalamate

Substance used to measure glomerular filtration rate for more accurate assessment of kidney function.

Glomeruli

The tiny filter units in each kidney that initiate the formation of urine. In health they allow only the liquid part of blood to be filtered, and a barrier against protein or cells like red blood cells appearing in the urine.

a serum creatinine concentration, the patient's age, gender, and ethnicity to a simple equation that would calculate the GFR while taking all these factors into consideration. In the appendix is a website that does this kind of calculation. For a sneak preview go to: www.kidney.org/professionals/KDOQI/gfr_calculator.cfm and enter the data given above and you will get a value of 69 mL/min/1.73m². The values above 60 mL/min/1.73m² are considered pretty good. Now, using the same website, change her creatinine value to 1.4 mg/dL, keeping in mind that this is still in the "normal" range. Her value is now 52. This, evident to even the most mathematically challenged among us, is less than 60 mL/min/1.73m² and is no longer in the "normal" range. This is why we began the answer to this question with a disclaimer regarding some of the difficulty involved in what is so straightforward a query.

The second part of this question is even more difficult to answer. A recent survey of doctors and patients suggests that very few patients, and not a whole lot of doctors, recognize when a person has a GFR less than 60 mL/min/1.73m², and is therefore not in the normal kidney function group. Candidly, some of the misconceptions arise from the fact that age is an important component of calculating GFR. Even though the creatinine level in your blood may not change between your 30th and your 65th birthday, your kidney function does change. Not convinced? If you are still at the website try using a value of 1.3, entering the age of 30, and then choosing your gender and appropriate ethnic category. Do the same thing but use the age of 65. Now you will begin to see some of the challenges in the classic Clinton response (forgive us here Bill . . .) "*define* kidney function." Our personal feeling as **nephrologists** is that it is reasonable to consider seeing a medical kidney doctor if your GFR is below 60 mL/min/1.73m². Keep in mind though that there are literally dozens of other times when referral to a medical kidney doctor is appropriate even with an absolutely normal GFR. We'll have more to say on that in later questions. We think that an even more appropriate referral to a medical kidney doctor is when the

Nephrologists

Physicians who specialize in the care of patients with kidney disease and hypertension.

change in kidney function exceeds that which we expect from normal aging. If you follow our logic and plug your numbers at age 30 and 65 into the website this would give you a fairly typical loss of kidney function with aging. This is not a strong reason to refer to a kidney doctor. It's usually a mixture of changing creatinine and other influences like protein in the urine that typically underlie a reason to send someone to a medical kidney doctor.

15. My doctor sent to me a kidney doctor who told me I have "stage 3 kidney disease." Can you explain what a stage is?

Building on our response to Question 14, we actually have to make a slight adjustment to our acronym GFR, to **eGFR**. This translates to *estimated* GFR. When you reread Question 14 where we introduced the GFR concept you'll see that the value the website is estimated from knowing four components: creatinine, age, ethnicity, and gender. When you plug these four values into a very tedious equation it estimates the GFR for you. Since it was estimated, and not actually measured by iothalamate, it is an eGFR. In the chart below, we show kidney function by the eGFR levels. We call these different categories stages of kidney function. There are five stages. You might wonder why we call stage one kidney disease since the kidney function is perfectly normal. This falls under the issue of what is "disease." Some people will have protein or blood in the urine and absolutely normal function and yet they have kidney disease. (Remember Question 10?) Some people have only one kidney, or have a kidney that looks funny on an X-ray or an ultrasound, and yet have perfectly normal function. In both of these instances there is evidence that something is not "perfectly normal" so the category of stage one kidney disease applies to people with good function but who have abnormalities in either the urine or the way the kidney appears when it is imaged. To answer this particular question, stage three kidney disease means that the eGFR is below 60 but higher than or equal to 30 mL/min/1.73m^2.

eGFR

Estimated GFR or glomerular filtration rate.

Table 2: National Kidney Foundation staging of chronic kidney disease

	eGFR value (mL/min/1.73m^2)	Approximate incidence in US adults (millions; see also figure 2)
Stage 1	≥ 90	6
Stage 2	60–89	5
Stage 3	30–59	7.5
Stage 4	15–29	<1
Stage 5	<15	<1

To calculate an eGFR go to: http://www.kidney.org/professionals/ KDOQI/gfr_calculator.cfm or get a very nerdy friend who is good at math and use the following formula:
eGFR = 175 × standardized serum creatinine − 1.154 × age − 0.203 × 1.212 [if black] × 0.742 [if female].
[Caveat: the creatinine should be stable for at least 3 months to use this formula.]

Cholesterol

A form of lipid important in heart disease. Cholesterol is the basis for sex hormones and bile, but it is also a substance that can accumulate in the lining of blood vessels and cause blockages.

In Figure 2, from a recent publication evaluating a random sample of adults in the United States, you can see that there are lots of people in the stage three kidney disease category. We mentioned previously that eGFR values below 60 represent reduced or abnormal kidney function. We think it's important to point out right here that there are virtually no symptoms that a person would experience in this range of kidney function (stage three). People don't tend to get sick from kidney disease until they are in stage five. The public health goal is to recognize people who are in stage three because we think that there are risks for progression to stage four or five. More importantly, the person's risks from cardiovascular disease like heart attack, heart failure, or stroke are higher than people whose kidney function is in an earlier stage. A lot of research is being conducted right now to better understand the nature of the increased risk for heart disease when kidney function falls into the stage three (or higher) category. It may be that common risk factors like high **cholesterol**, elevated

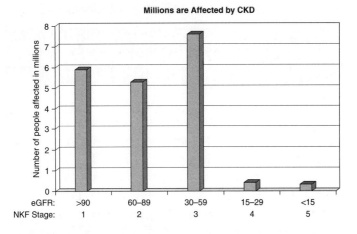

Figure 2. NKF staging system and number of people with CKD based on the eGFR value.

blood sugar, being overweight, etc., are just more frequent or more potent as risk factors when a person is in stage three (or higher) category.

Both authors of this book are involved in the CRIC study (www.cristudy.org) that specifically addresses questions like this, so we are hopeful that edition two of this book will have more information on the mechanisms associated with cardiovascular risk.

16. My doctor said my GFR is reduced. What does that mean?

As we mentioned previously, most people who have stage three kidney disease (see Question 15) have no symptoms and so are unaware that they are at this level of kidney function. They find out only if a doctor orders a blood test. In the past few years, several states have required the laboratory performing the serum creatinine measurement to report the eGFR on the lab slip. Consequently, the number of times a person's reduced GFR is recognized is on the rise.

Now, to address the question. What a reduced GFR means is that your level of creatinine relative to your age, gender and ethnicity is in a range that is statistically abnormal. That's the first part of the answer to this question. The more important part is: What does it mean?

There are two principal consequences. The first is that your chances of losing more kidney function are higher because kidney function is already compromised. This means that the remaining filter units in your kidney have to work that much harder to do the daily job of getting rid of the waste products. Think of yourself as working in a factory with a hundred people. Times are tough, there is a persistent demand for the product, but people are not willing to pay as much. Management decides to lay off 50 percent of the workforce. This means the remaining 50 percent have to do 100 percent of the work in order to maintain production. The same thing happens with your kidneys as function is lost. Since a normal GFR is about 100 mL/min/1.73m^2, when the GFR drops to 50 mL/min/1.73m^2 the filter units that remain have to work twice as hard to get rid of the daily waste. How long do you think you can go working daily 16-hour shifts? That's the question that faces your kidneys. For reasons that we don't quite understand, oftentimes the kidneys do just fine and last for many years even with reduced function. Other people, by contrast, have a much more rapid loss of function.

One other thing to mention at this point is that reduced kidney function sometimes determines dosing of medications.

The second consequence is that you are at greater risk for heart disease and stroke. As we mentioned in Question 15, the reasons for that are still being researched. In the meantime, our advice is to take a careful look at the things you can fix such as blood pressure and the other items we mentioned previously. More attention to detail is the goal here since the cardiovascular risks are higher.

One other thing to mention at this point is that reduced kidney function sometimes determines dosing of medications.

Many drugs are excreted by the kidney and reduce levels of kidney function, which means that less drug goes a longer way. Doctors have access to a resource called the Physicians' Desk Reference (which is also available online at www.pdr.net, but you'll need to register) that provides details for dosing drugs based upon kidney function.

Finally, there isn't much we can do to recover lost kidney function. The most important thing is to maximize our efforts at preserving residual function for as long as possible. It is in this area that nephrologists have much to offer and can add to the efforts of general practice physicians in achieving this goal.

17. When should a patient with abnormal kidney function see a kidney specialist? Can my primary care physician take care of this problem?

We have skirted around this issue on several previous questions and now it's time to take it head on. Sometimes, a patient is not referred to a kidney specialist until his or her kidney function loss is so advanced that they are **uremic**. At this point the kidney doctor can do little more than console the patient on their loss of kidney function and start them on dialysis while considering whether or not they are a transplant candidate. This is too late for the referral to a kidney specialist.

When the authors look at their own profiles of patients, we believe that the best time to refer a patient to a kidney specialist is under the following circumstances:

1. When there is an abnormality in the urine or an unexplained reduction in kidney function.

2. When there is comorbidity present, like diabetes, and there are early changes in kidney function that worry the primary care doctor.

Uremic

Showing symptoms of nausea, vomiting, weight loss, decreased appetite, and fatigue associated with renal failure that is severe enough to consider starting dialysis.

3. When the primary care physician feels out of his or her league in managing this aspect of the patient's care.

4. When there are changes in blood tests that suggest that kidney function may be taking a toll on other aspects of health that require intimate knowledge of drugs that primary care physicians don't commonly use. For example, fancy versions of vitamin D or injectable medications that stimulate red blood cell production.

From the guidelines standpoint, the National Kidney Foundation has a couple of recommendations to offer, as well. These are found at the National Kidney Foundation Kidney Disease Outcomes Quality Initiative website which is cited in the appendix. What they say is:

"Patients with mild decreased GFR, low risk for progressive decline in GFR, and low risk for cardiovascular disease have a good prognosis and may require only adjustment of the dosage of drugs that are excreted by the kidney, monitoring of blood pressure, avoidance of drugs and procedures with risk for acute kidney failure, and life-style modifications to reduce the risk of cardiovascular disease. Consultation with the nephrologist may be necessary to establish the diagnosis and treatment of the type of kidney disease. Kidney function should be monitored at least yearly.

Patients with moderately or severely decreased GFR or risk factors for faster decline in GFR or cardiovascular disease have a worse prognosis. In addition to the interventions mentioned above, they require assessment for complications of decreased GFR and dietary and pharmacologic therapy directed at slowing the progression of kidney disease and ameliorating cardiovascular risk factor levels. Consultation and/or co-management with a kidney disease care team is advisable during stage three, and referral to a nephrologist in stage four is recommended. Kidney function may need to be monitored four times per year or more. A multidisciplinary team approach may be necessary to implement and coordinate care.

As to whether your primary care physician can manage your care, the answer is "sometimes." It has to do with the comfort level of the primary care physician, their experience managing such patients, and, in some cases, the ease of communication with nephrologists who sometimes share office space in the same building. Not uncommonly, doctors chat with one another about patient care problems in what we call a "curbside consult." Both authors have frequently given advice about patient management when there is a simple question present and no need for a formal referral. In some cases a curbside consult is not possible and at that point we recommend formal referral.

David's comments:

As Dr. Townsend and Dr. Cohen stated, the patient usually doesn't get a handle on a potential problem until late. I am of the firm conviction that if you suffer from diabetes, you should make an appointment to see a renal specialist. Especially, if you are suffering vision problems. Vision problems and kidney problems usually go hand in hand in diabetics. Dr. Cohen got my blood pressure under control along with my proteinuria. This dramatically slows down the disease's progress. Relying on a primary care physician to treat kidney disease is just not enough. You need a dedicated team— including a nutritionist.

18. I had an ultrasound today of my kidneys. What can my doctor learn from an ultrasound?

Lots. We *love* ultrasounds and recommend them to all our friends! They don't hurt, are typically without risk, patients rarely refuse having them done again, and they provide great information. To be sure, they have limits but they can tell us several very important things that factor into the evaluation and management of patients with kidney issues. The first thing they tell us is how many kidneys you have.

Most people have two. Some people were born with one kidney, and some people have lost the function of one kidney over time because of trauma, infection, or things like kidney stone disease. In some cases one kidney has been removed. It's useful to know this information, especially if someone has only one kidney. Needless to say, they would make a poor kidney donor should a family member be on dialysis and in need of a kidney. Rarely, some people have three kidneys, and some people have a kidney that looks like a horseshoe because the bottoms of each kidney are physically connected together in the midline just in front of the spine.

Ultrasounds tell us the kidney sizes. This helps us to understand whether reduced kidney function is chronic, in which case the kidneys are usually on the small side, or acute, in which case the kidney sizes may be normal, or even enlarged.

Ultrasounds tell us whether the flow of urine out of the kidney into the collecting system is normal or obstructed. This can be very important information in understanding a sudden reduction in kidney function. This could occur, for example, if the **prostate** gland enlarges to the point of blocking flow out of the bladder, which in turn backs up the collecting system to the kidney. In this situation, one or both kidneys may show dilation in the collecting system because of the backup.

Prostate

The prostate is an exocrine gland of the male mammalian reproductive system.

Ultrasounds may tell us whether there are kidney stones present. See Question 83 for more information.

Finally, an ultrasound may show abnormalities such as tumors, scars, and other things in one or both kidneys that might explain things like blood in the urine. All of these things are important in the evaluation and management of people who have issues with either kidney function, changes in blood or urine tests related to the kidneys, or things like flank pain that may be associated with the problem in the flow of urine from the kidney to the bladder.

19. My kidney doctor seemed concerned because there were casts in my urine. What are casts?

To answer this question we're going to need to do a little bit of Kidney Anatomy 101. Figure 3 will help in this regard. This figure shows the basic unit into which our kidneys are divided, which is called the nephron.

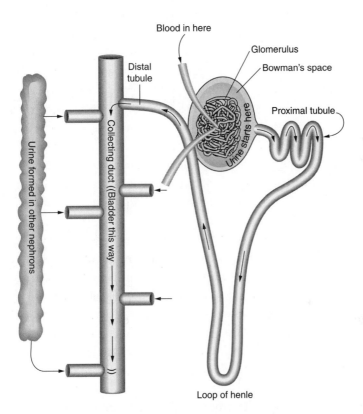

Blood in here

Glomerulus

Distal tubule

Bowman's space

Proximal tubule

Collecting duct ((Bladder this way

Urine starts here

Urine formed in other nephrons

Loop of henle

Figure 3: The Nephron. Urine formation starts in the Bowman's space after blood is filtered in the Glomerulus. The filtered blood (now called urine) travels along the tubules (with most of the water and important salts re-absorbed along the way) until it reaches the Collecting Duct, where it will make its way out of the kidney, into the ureters and collect in the bladder (resulting in that familiar sensation known as "urgency" when ignored for too long).

Glomerulus

These are the tiny filter units in each kidney that initiate the formation of urine. In health they allow only the liquid part of blood to be filtered, and a barrier against protein or cells like red blood cells appearing in the urine.

Bowman's space

The space surrounding the glomerulus of each nephron or kidney "filter" unit.

Crystal

Precipitate that is seen under a microscope when looking at the urine in a patient with kidney stones.

At the front end is the **glomerulus** from Question 14. Blood is filtered at this point and becomes filtrate just beyond the glomerulus, in the region called **Bowman's space**. The filtrate travels from Bowman's space into the tubular system. The tubular system is divided into a front end, called the proximal tubule, and the back end called the distal tubule. Just as all roads lead to Rome, all distal tubules lead to collecting ducts. The collecting ducts are the conduits by which urine is passed from the kidney into the beginning of the collecting system. To understand what a cast is and how it is formed consider the following: What happens when you drip vinegar on an egg white? No need to run to the fridge to find this one out, let us tell you instead (its lots less messy this way). When you mix the acetic acid in vinegar with the albumin in the egg white it forms a cloudy white substance called a coagulum. The clear egg white now turns to a cloudy or opaque white color because the acid has caused the proteins in the egg white, which were previously in solution, to precipitate. The same thing happens when rain becomes snow. The water molecules in the clear raindrops are in solution. When they form a **crystal**, they are white and opaque. The proteins in the egg white when they are in solution let you see through the egg white. When you precipitate them, or crystallize them with the acetic acid, they form the coagulum. This is basically what happens when protein present in the kidney tubule meets up with acid secreted by the tubule cells. This secreted acid causes the protein in the tubule to precipitate, just like the egg white when exposed to vinegar. Because the tubule is round and long like a pipe, the protein that precipitates takes all in the cylindrical shape of the tubule. The buildup of urine behind it pushes the precipitated protein down the tubule and out into the urine that collects in the bladder ultimately. We call the precipitated protein a cast because, like in pottery, it is a cast of the tubule lining.

In situations where we are a little deprived of fluid (like a 2K run, for example), there are normally a few casts in the urine.

The protein that forms these casts is actually made in the kidney itself. These casts are otherwise devoid of things like blood cells that happened to be there abnormally when the cast was formed. Such casts look kind of empty and are called hyaline casts. Hyaline casts are usually thought to have no significance. When casts form around cells like red or white blood cells, these casts are far more important and lead us to consider damage in the filter units (the glomeruli) or damage to the kidney tissue itself from infection or **inflammation**. In patients who are in the hospital, and usually pretty sick, there are times when some of the medications that are used, some of the tests that use contrast media or dye, or specific things like serious infection cause an abrupt loss of kidney function. In these situations the whole tubule actually ends up decomposing and has granular or grainy appearance in a cast in the urine. Sometimes casts are a sign that a serious insult to kidney function has occurred, but this is usually in hospitalized patients.

As with everything that can be associated with the kidneys, we try to keep a perspective on all the findings a patient has. When we find casts in the urine we ask ourselves whether such findings are consistent with other tests, with the patient's history, with other disorders that may be present, etc. In some cases, the presence of red cell casts in particular leads us to recommend tests such as a **kidney biopsy** in selected patients. Consequently, the type of cast matters in terms of what we do after we find casts are present.

20. My doctor says I need a kidney biopsy. What does that involve? Will it help find the cause for my kidney disease?

A kidney biopsy is undertaken when we think it's really important to understand the specific cause of a finding in the urine or blood that indicates a serious disease is present in the kidney.

Inflammation

The ability of a hormone, or a germ like a bacteria or virus, or some other influence to cause a reaction in the body that involves some aspect of the immune system. The result of this reaction is often a buildup of scar or plaque. Inflammation is thought to play a big role in hardening of the arteries.

Kidney biopsy

A procedure usually performed with ultrasound guidance to obtain a small piece or core of kidney tissue which is then examined under a microscope to assess the cause of a patient's kidney disease.

Lupus (SLE)

A chronic generalized connective tissue disorder, ranging from mild to fulminating, marked by skin eruptions, arthralgia, arthritis, leukopenia, anemia, visceral lesions, neurologic manifestations, lymphadenopathy, fever, and other constitutional symptoms.

A kidney biopsy is undertaken when we think it's really important to understand the specific cause of a finding in the urine or blood that indicates a serious disease is present in the kidney.

Some kidney diseases are treatable, but the therapies are often somewhat toxic. This means that we need to feel that the risks of treatment are not outweighed by the potential benefits of improving kidney function, or kidney inflammation from specific diseases such as **lupus**. A kidney biopsy involves several steps. It's usually done in conjunction with a radiologist, though some nephrologists are trained in ultrasound and can locate the kidneys without the need for a radiologist. The first step is to verify that two kidneys are present and to decide which one to biopsy. As we mentioned previously, the kidneys are tucked up under the ribs so the patient has to take and hold a deep breath to bring the kidneys down below the level of the last rib making them accessible for the biopsy procedure.

When we are ready to biopsy, the patient lies on their stomach, the skin is prepped with an antibiotic solution to minimize the chance of causing an infection from the process, then we numb the skin with an anesthetic. There is little in the way of nerves between the skin and the kidney so most of our effort is to numb the skin. Next, we make a tiny incision to allow insertion of the biopsy needle. The incision is about an eighth of an inch and does not need a suture. Then we insert a long thin needle down to the surface of the kidney. We ask the patient to take a deep breath and hold it. Once the breath is held, we press the trigger on the biopsy needle apparatus, and a tiny sliver of kidney tissue is captured in the tip of the needle. It's about the size of a very thin spaghetti noodle. Our biopsy core is smaller than the spaghetti noodle in diameter and typically a quarter to a half-inch long. Typically, two or three passes are made with the biopsy needle to obtain enough tissue to do all the testing necessary.

Most of the time, the biopsy will find the cause for kidney disease. There are a couple of situations where the biopsy may not tell us what's wrong. This can happen when we biopsy an area of the kidney that is so damaged that all we see is a scar. Scar is the end result of the damage, but doesn't tell us what it was, exactly, that caused the damage in the first place. Some kidney diseases do not affect all the kidney tissue to the same degree. Some diseases are more focal as opposed to diffuse, and sampling error means that the 10 or so glomeruli that we obtained from the biopsy did not show the disease process. Keep in mind that you have on average one million glomeruli in each kidney. If half of them are affected and half or not, and we remove only 10, sometimes we miss diseases that are affecting the kidney because the 10 glomeruli we obtained were all from the half that do not show the disease. Finally, the biopsy may show us that the kidneys are inflamed, for example, but give us no clue as to what was causing the inflammation. Bear in mind that these are exceptions and not the rule. Most times when nephrologists undertake a kidney biopsy, it is for a specific reason, often related to anticipated treatment decisions. The biopsy helps inform greatly the choice of what to do. Sometimes, a biopsy is undertaken in a patient who had a previous biopsy because of an unanticipated or unexpected result in the course of treatment.

Biopsies are something that nephrologists do only with much thought given before recommending it. The reason nephrologists are so cautious is that the kidney has more blood vessels than virtually any other organ in the body. Consequently, the biggest risk from a kidney biopsy is bleeding. One hundred percent of the time bleeding occurs after a biopsy and it occurs deep within the body because the kidneys are several inches underneath the skin. Fortunately, the bleeding is almost always self-contained and stops on its own.

David's comments:

I am told a kidney biopsy usually doesn't reveal the nature rather it eliminates some potential causes.

21. I have been diagnosed with kidney disease. Can I become pregnant and, if I do, will it make my kidney disease worse?

This is an important question. When you think about what the mother's kidneys do during gestation, they have to do double duty particularly as the forming fetus approaches the size of the newborn. There is a pretty impressive series of adaptations that occur in the normal kidneys when a woman becomes pregnant. The kidneys become a little larger, and their function as measured by blood tests appears to be supernormal. We mentioned previously that a normal serum creatinine concentration in most laboratories is between 0.5 to 1.5 mg/dL. The normal serum creatinine concentration during pregnancy is about 0.4 to 0.6 mg/dL. These changes in kidney function occur from a number of sources of hormonal changes and other signals that adapt the kidney to the requirements that the **gravid** state necessitates.

Gravid

Pregnant state.

Multidisciplinary team

A team approach often involving a few different physicians, nurses, dietitian, social worker, and other health care workers who all work together to come up with and implement a treatment management plan.

There are some data that give us a clue as to what happens to kidney function during pregnancy in women with pre-existing kidney disease. In general, the news is not good. Contemplating having a child with reduced kidney function is a big deal, and requires a **multidisciplinary team** consisting of a high risk obstetrician, the nephrologist, perhaps an endocrinologist as well as the primary care doctor. The type of kidney disease and the severity of function loss are very important considerations in answering this question. When the reduction in kidney function is minor and due, for example, to prior self-limited damage such as an episode of severe kidney infection, the kidneys may fare better during pregnancy than if you have something such as type 1 diabetes affecting your kidneys where the kidney function is down in the 20 percent of normal range, or in stage four as we mentioned previously in Question 15 and show in Table 2. Because of an interesting quirk, the GFR and percentage of normal kidney function are virtually identical numbers. So when we say that kidney function is 20 percent of normal we are pretty close to a GFR of 20 mL/min/1.73m². In addition, a very key issue to consider is the presence of protein in the urine and the amount of protein, if present. Even in normal pregnancies, urine protein excretion about doubles. In a patient with pre-existing proteinuria who becomes pregnant, the increased loss of protein in the urine can be really large. This generates a problem for how the body handles fluids. The loss of excessive protein through the urine causes the body to signal the kidneys to retain salt, which causes a build-up of excess salt and water in the legs, abdomen, and the pleural space.

The other part of this question has to do with the word "can." In some cases, the disorders leading to reduced kidney function also exact a toll on the function of the ovaries and uterus. Sometimes women with **chronic kidney diseases** lose their normal periods. In such cases, achieving pregnancy can be quite difficult, though not always impossible.

The disorder called **preeclampsia** is more common in patients when they have pre-existing kidney function reduction. Preeclampsia is characterized by urine protein losses that are elevated, increasing blood pressure, further reductions in kidney function, and changes in blood tests including those of the liver enzymes and the platelet levels. All of these things need to be taken into account when counseling a woman with kidney disease regarding the advisability of pregnancy.

Chronic kidney disease

Longstanding damage to the kidneys or chronic kidney failure.

Preeclampsia

A situation, usually arising after the 20th week of pregnancy, characterized by increased blood pressure, ankle swelling, and proteinuria in a pregnant woman.

22. If I still pass a lot of urine does this mean my kidney function is still good?

Though we wish we could assure you that passage of urine is equivalent with good function of the kidney, the fact is that the two are not at all so well related. Let us give an example. There are many patients on kidney dialysis who pass a perfectly normal amount of urine in the course of the day. How can this be?

Some basic math will help shed some light here. Let's go back to our GFR for just a minute. We said that the normal value is about 100 mL/min/1.73m^2 and then through all those gobbledygook letters after it. It's time to unpack what those letters mean. For reference here's what they were: mL/min/1.73m^2. The two parts of this that are important are:

1. the letters "mL" which stands for milliliters and
2. the letters "min" which abbreviate the word minute.

It takes 1,000 mL to make a liter which is roughly equal in size to a quart. So if we do some quick math calculations, every 10 minutes the kidneys filter a quart of fluid from the blood. Remember your high school algebra? Take a look at this equation and you'll see how it works:

$$100 \text{ mL/min} \times 10 \text{ min} = 1{,}000 \text{ mL}$$

This means that every hour our kidneys make 6 liters (or about 6 quarts) of filtrate that can ultimately become urine. Multiply that times 24 hours since our kidneys never get a vacation, and you'll see that they make about 140 liters (or quarts) of filtrate per day. They reabsorbed about 99 percent of the filtrate so that only one or two liters actually become urine. When kidney function is reduced 50 percent, kidneys still make 70 liters of filtrate per day. They reabsorbed 97 percent and you still have 1 or 2 liters of urine. Even if you reduce your kidney function to 5 percent of normal, a huge reduction by anyone's estimate, the kidneys are still filtering approximately 8 liters per day. If they've reabsorbed three quarters of this, that still leaves room for 2 liters of urine to be made and voided.

The converse, however, that no urine production means that kidney function is reduced is much more likely to be true. There are dialysis patients who make no urine. There are also very sick patients in the hospital whose urine output is very low or nonexistent, and this usually has reduced kidney function with it.

Moral of story: you can't judge kidney function by the quantity of urine produced. You can only tell function when you actually measure it with blood tests.

PART THREE

Hypertension and Kidney Disease

How common is high blood pressure (hypertension) in people with kidney disease?

Are there special medicines for high blood pressure when I have kidney disease?

My doctor was concerned that my kidney arteries are blocked. Why would she think that?

More . . .

Hypertension

Also called high blood pressure. Hypertension is a circumstance in which a person's blood pressure has been shown to be consistently at or above 140/90 mm Hg. Hypertension is a leading risk factor for stroke, heart disease, kidney disease, and peripheral circulation problems.

Diabetic nephropathy

Chronic kidney disease due to diabetes.

Interstitium

The supporting tissue of the kidney.

23. How common is high blood pressure (hypertension) in people with kidney disease?

Pretty common. Much more common than in the general population. One place that has systematically evaluated the prevalence of **hypertension** is the CRIC study we mentioned previously in Question 15. In the CRIC study, hypertension was present in about 85 percent of all the subjects enrolled in our study. We have about 3,600 such folks and roughly half have diabetes. The reason we mention the diabetes aspect is that this particular form of kidney disease, which we called **diabetic nephropathy**, almost always has high blood pressure present. There are some chronic kidney diseases where kidney function is reduced and yet blood pressure is conspicuously normal. These types of diseases tend to not so much affect the glomeruli primarily, but attack the supporting tissue of the kidney which is called the **interstitium**. In such situations, the kidney sometimes actually loses sodium and the blood pressure can be on the low side. These are, however, less common as the cause of reduced kidney function.

The importance of blood pressure in kidney disease cannot be stressed enough. It seems to be a crucial component of the progression of kidney disease when it is inadequately treated. The problem is that sometimes the blood pressure increase causes the kidney disease, and sometimes the blood pressure increase is the result of the damage to the kidney itself. We say in the situation that the kidney is both the victim and the villain when it comes to high blood pressure.

As with reduced kidney function, once again there is little in the way of specific symptoms that point to the presence of elevated blood pressure. Therefore we strongly urge, recommend, insist, and endorse unequivocally having your blood pressure checked *regularly* if your kidney function is reduced, or if you have been told you have "kidney disease." Elevated levels of blood pressure are one of the few things that you can correct in the process of doing everything possible to preserve residual kidney function.

David's comments:

As a member of the CRIC study group, a heavy emphasis was placed on hypertension. The CRIC study is the most comprehensive and groundbreaking study that has ever been focused on the kidney. If there was one thing I gleaned from being involved with the study, it's the distinct relationship between hypertension and kidney disease.

24. Why are people with kidney disease so prone to high blood pressure?

This is a great question. The connection between high blood pressure and kidney disease has been known for more than a century. What is it about the kidneys that predisposes a person to elevated blood pressure when their function is impaired? To answer this we need to do a little bit of kidney physiology and then take those findings and piece them back into the ultimate control of blood pressure. Let's start with the diagram in Figure 4.

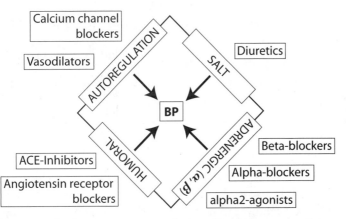

Figure 4. Blood pressure servos and where blood pressure medicines work.

This diagram shows the 4 main influences on blood pressure. "Adrenergic" refers to the sympathetic nervous system. "Humoral" refers to things that circulate like hormones. "Autoregulation" refers to what blood vessels can do, on their own, when the other influences on blood pressure are removed. Boxes show where medicines work.

From *100 Questions and Answers About High Blood Pressure (Hypertension)*, Raymond Townsend MD, Jones and Bartlett Publishers, LLC © 2008.

Let's start with the salt. There really is only one system, one organ that is able to govern the salt levels in the body. Whether you crave salt, or whether you avoid it like the plague, you can't get away from it. There is a bit of sodium, the active principle in salt, in virtually all foods except distilled water and rice. Most fruits, too, are relatively low in sodium. This finding was leveraged in the 1940s by Walter Kempner at Duke University who championed the use of the "rice and fruit diet" in the management of high blood pressure at a time when there were virtually no blood pressure medications available. What he found was that if you can reduce drastically the amount of sodium, in particular sodium chloride, that a person consumes in their diet you can make a difference in blood pressure. The problem was the stringent nature of the diet itself. At the time, the choice was between the diet or death from heart failure or stroke. You can see why people chose the diet. When kidney function is damaged, the ability of the kidneys to excrete the daily salt intake can suffer. One of the compensations for this reduced ability to get rid of the daily salt load, is to elevate the blood pressure. Think of it in a mechanical way. As the blood pressure goes up, the force behind the glomerular filtration rate increases since the blood pressure is what drives blood into the glomeruli in the first place. We call this kind of pressure "hydraulic" meaning it's related to the force behind the fluid. If the increase in blood pressure was all that was needed to force more salt into the urine by virtue of whipping the glomeruli into more filtration, and there was no consequence to that, we wouldn't be having this discussion now. The problem, of course, is that the elevated blood pressure doesn't just do this glomerular thing. It strains the heart, the brain, and other tissues in the process. These other organs experience something we would colloquially call "collateral damage." Consequently, it's important to control the blood pressure not just for the sake of the heart and brain, but because the elevated blood pressure also takes a toll on the residual kidney function.

Insulin

A hormone produced in the pancreas that regulates the amount of sugar in the blood by stimulating cells, especially liver and muscle cells, to absorb and metabolize glucose. Insulin also stimulates the conversion of blood glucose into glycogen and fat, which are the body's chief sources of stored carbohydrates

Next you see side of the diagram that's labeled "humoral." Humors is a synonym for hormones and other chemicals that circulate in the blood and travel from tissue to tissue accomplishing some purpose. **Insulin** is a humor, or a hormone, made by the pancreas which travels in the blood to places like the liver to promote the uptake of sugar from the blood and its storage in that organ. The kidney is important when it comes to humors. It generates **renin**, one of the most important humors that control blood pressure. You can get a sense of how important this particular hormone is by recognizing that the three different classes of blood pressure medications specifically attack different aspects of the renin system. These blood pressure medicines are called angiotensin-converting enzyme inhibitors, angiotensin **receptor** blockers, and direct renin inhibitors. The kidney is the principal source of the renin found in the blood. As kidneys fail, it would make sense to stop making renin since that only contributes to higher blood pressure in a vicious cycle. However, renin is normally made and released as a defense against blood loss. As they fail, the kidneys sometimes react as though they're not getting enough blood, which leads to the generation of the excessive renin.

Furthermore, the kidneys actually play a role in the activity of the involuntary nervous system. When kidneys fail, the **sympathetic** side of the involuntary nervous system becomes more active. This is the part of the involuntary nervous system that drives up blood pressure and heart rate. It's not clear *how* this happens, but it is pretty clear *that* it does happen. Increased activity of the sympathetic nervous system is an important part of the hypertension that is so common in kidney disease.

Finally, the fourth side of the diagram looks at the blood vessel itself, apart from all these other things. If you were to greatly enlarge your average blood vessel, you would see that it has three layers. The innermost layer is just one cell thick and is called the **endothelium**. This innermost layer has been the source of much research over the last 20 years including a Nobel Prize given to researchers who discovered that the

Renin

A circulating enzyme released mainly by juxtaglomerular cells in the juxtaglomerular apparatus of the kidneys in response to low blood volume.

Receptor

This term usually refers to a protein that is anchored on the surface of a cell that specifically attracts a certain chemical or hormone.

Sympathetic

Part of the involuntary nervous system that increases heart rate and increases blood pressure.

Endothelium

A thin layer of flat epithelial cells that lines the lymph vessels, blood vessels, and the inner cavities of the heart.

The muscle portion of the wall is the thickest and it's the part that generates the blood pressure.

Angiotensin-converting enzyme (ACE) inhibitors

A commonly used drug that blocks the renin angiotensin system. These drugs are used to lower blood pressure and decrease protein in the urine.

Angiotensin receptor blocker (ARB)

Another commonly used drug that blocks the renin angiotensin system at a different receptor. ARBs are a type of blood pressure medication that also reduces protein in the urine and are commonly used in patients with diabetic kidney disease.

Direct renin inhibitors

A new class of drugs that inhibit renin and are also used for the treatment of high blood pressure.

endothelium makes a substance that promotes relaxation of the muscle portion of the blood vessel wall. The muscle portion of the wall is the thickest and it's the part that generates the blood pressure. The outermost layer is called the adventitia and we are mostly clueless about what the adventitia does. When kidney function is reduced, things begin to build up in the blood, interfering with the substance made by the endothelium that promotes relaxation in the muscular wall component of the blood vessel.

You now see how important the kidney is to all the things that govern blood pressure. Salt, humors, the involuntary nervous system, and the nature of the blood vessel itself all are affected when kidney function declines. This is why high blood pressure is so common as kidneys fail.

David's comments:

My doctor, Debbie Cohen, had success in lowering my proteinuria with an ace-inhibitor called lisinopril.

25. Are there special medicines for high blood pressure when I have kidney disease?

The answer to this question depends somewhat on the nature of the disease damaging the kidney function. For example, the most common is diabetes. When diabetes affects the kidneys, there is usually a significant amount of protein present in the urine. The class of blood pressure medicines called **angiotensin-converting enzyme (ACE) inhibitors** and the class of blood pressure medicines called **angiotensin receptor blockers** have both been used in treating the blood pressure elevation in patients with kidney disease and diabetes. They have been shown to preserve kidney function better than other drug classes that lower blood pressure to the same degree. The newer class of blood pressure medicines called the **direct renin inhibitors** will probably fall into this category as well, but the research is not complete enough at this time to say for certain.

When people have kidney disease that it is not characterized by large amounts of protein in the urine, there is little information to suggest that one class of blood pressure medications is more effective than another in either reducing their blood pressure or preserving their kidney function. In that situation, the goal is to get the blood pressure down by whatever means.

Reconsidering Question 24, it makes sense that getting blood pressure under control in a patient who has kidney function impairment is often a substantial challenge requiring several classes of antihypertensive drugs to be used. Typically, it takes at least three classes of drugs to get the blood pressure under control.

From time to time there have been news reports and research studies indicating that sometimes blood pressure medicines can make certain aspects of kidney disease worse. For example, the class of medications called calcium channel blockers when used alone in patients who have protein in the urine can sometimes (depending on the particular calcium channel blocker used) make the protein losses higher even though the blood pressure has been reduced. This provides a mixed benefit. Our goal is typically to lower the blood pressure *and* to lower the urinary protein losses. When we lower blood pressure but increase urine protein losses, we may not preserve kidney function as well. The lesson here is that our goal in treating high blood pressure in patients with kidney disease is always keeping in sight the effect our treatment is having—not just on the blood pressure, but on things like urine protein losses.

Finally, it sometimes happens that kidney function gets worse as blood pressure is reduced. This sometimes scares patients a great deal. Consider this: if your kidneys are working overtime to clear your blood of waste, and you use a medication that reduces their workload, as measured by a reduction in their GFR, this might be good in some situations. We use a term called "**hyperfiltration**" to characterize the overworked kidneys. This is a complicated concept but in a nutshell it says that

Hyperfiltration

A condition where the kidney has increased processing of fluids through the kidney.

Hypertension and Kidney Disease

41

the kidneys are adapting to reduced function by working their individual glomeruli at, for example, 150 percent of normal. If we believe that the magnitude of this overload contributes to the loss of the remaining glomeruli that are working so hard to clear the blood, then undoing some of the hyperfiltration forces by a specific drug treatment may actually be a good thing if we're willing to sacrifice a short-term loss in function for a long term slowing of the rate of loss in the rest of the kidney. Look at the graph below in Figure 5. In one line you see the effects of doing nothing and the ultimate loss of kidney function to the point of requiring dialysis or a transplant. In another line, you see a greater loss in the short term but an alteration in the slope of the line such that it takes a longer period until kidney function is lost to the point of requiring dialysis or a transplant. This is the subtle balance that nephrologists always weigh in our decisions of what to use to manage the blood pressure in a patient whose kidney function is impaired.

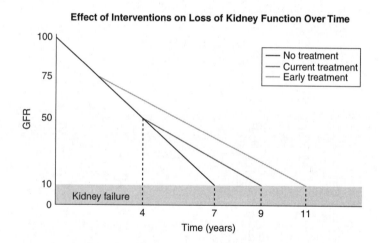

Effect of Interventions on Loss of Kidney Function Over Time

Figure 5. Effect of interventions on loss of kidney function over time. The straight dark line is the loss of kidney function over time in the 4 years before and following recognition. Treatment at the time of discovery (4 years) can slow down the loss of function, but earlier recognition and treatment (the upper line) is best.

26. I thought my blood pressure was pretty good when it registered 134/84 mm Hg in the doctor's office, but she told me it should be even lower than that. Why is that?

No doubt you've heard of the Holy Grail or, more importantly, the search for the Holy Grail (Monty Python notwithstanding). In some ways, defining the best blood pressure, which we call the blood pressure goal, has been like the search for the Holy Grail. Until approximately 15 years ago, we didn't have a clue about what the best blood pressure should be in patients with kidney disease. Moreover, achieving blood pressure goals lower than that of the blood pressure in the question itself (134/84 mm Hg) usually requires a substantial amount of medication in a patient very dedicated to taking the medication. At the time of this writing, the blood pressure goal for someone diagnosed with hypertension and chronic kidney disease (or diabetes, or heart disease) is 130/80 mm Hg. You might wonder how we arrived at that number. Moreover, you might be aware that the typical definition of hypertension is a blood pressure of equal to or more than 140 mm Hg for the upper number and equal to or more than 90 mm Hg for the lower number. Both the upper number and the lower number matter in determining hypertension. A person with a blood pressure 142/78 mm Hg has hypertension and a person with 126/94 mm Hg has hypertension. Part of the confusion is that we still define "hypertension" as 140/90 mm Hg even if kidney disease is present. However, the treatment goal is less than 130/80 mm Hg once we diagnose hypertension in people with chronic kidney disease. We still haven't answered the question where did the 130/80 come from?

Our guidelines were prepared by agencies like the National Kidney Foundation who have sifted through the available information from treating high blood pressure in large **clinical trials** over the past 40 years. When they tabulated the existing data and looked in particular at the degree of blood

Clinical trials

A group of people with a finding (like hypertension) are randomly assigned one or another treatment (usually without the nature of the treatment being known to the doctors conducting the study or the patients taking the treatment: this is called "blinding") and followed for a long time to see if one treatment has better outcomes (like less strokes, for example) compared with the other treatment.

Hypertension and Kidney Disease

pressure reduction and the loss of kidney function with time, it is the impression of these agencies that the 140/90 mm Hg goal, while fine for most uncomplicated hypertensives, needed refinement for those with chronic kidney disease.

The evidence is strongest for those with diabetes. The evidence is pretty strong in those that have large amounts of protein in the urine. In particular for those who have more than 1 g of protein lost in the urine each day. For those who simply have reduced kidney function but are not diabetic nor do they have significant proteinuria, the evidence is less strong. The argument for the 130/80 mm Hg goal in this latter category is based upon reasoning that the heart and the brain still benefit from the lower degrees of blood pressure even though evidence proving that such a stringent degree of blood pressure reduction (again in the absence of diabetes or significant proteinuria) preserves kidney function is still lacking. The issue in the absence of diabetes or significant proteinuria is whether 130/80 mm Hg is better than 140/90 mm Hg as a treatment goal to preserve kidney function. We just don't have evidence to prove that at this time. The answer to this question is that the guidelines strongly suggest 130/80 mm Hg without doing all the nitpicking we have done in answering this question. Hopefully, by the time this question is addressed again, perhaps in five years, we'll have more information.

27. If I have high blood pressure, can I safely have a pregnancy? Are there any risks to myself or the baby?

This question expands one we covered previously regarding pregnancy in chronic kidney disease. Taking the first part of this question, the answer is yes. Many women with high blood pressure are able to safely **conceive** and carry to term. It is, however, not a cakewalk to accomplish this and requires close networking with a team dedicated to managing all the aspects and potential problems that a pregnancy complicated by hypertension can engender.

Many women with high blood pressure are able to safely conceive and carry to term.

Conceive

When a female becomes pregnant.

The first issue is how to control the blood pressure during pregnancy. This also addresses some of the second part of this question. During pregnancy, the risks to the mother carrying the child are largely related to the vulnerability of target organs, like the brain, to high blood pressure, which seems to be increased when pregnancy is present. The damage high blood pressure can do to target organs is enhanced at any level of blood pressure compared to those who are not pregnant. We can usually manage pregnancy-related hypertension effectively and provide optimal safety to the mother and the child. The key issue is to recognize the potential risks, especially those that practitioners may cause by use of certain medications.

There are a few other risks to the mother. We talked a bit about preeclampsia in Question 21. Some other things to consider are worsening of kidney function and worsening of urinary protein losses.

There are also risks to the baby, including being small for **gestational** age, or predisposed to potential birth defects because of exposure to certain blood pressure drugs. A large experiment from the state of Tennessee involving more than 29,000 babies and their mothers underscores some of this concern. In that study, mothers who took ACE inhibitors at any point during pregnancy had babies with higher rates of birth defects. The results were reported in the *New England Journal of Medicine* in June 2006 and this is what the investigators reported in their study:

Gestational

Having to do with pregnancy.

"Infants with only first-trimester exposure to ACE inhibitors had an increased risk of major congenital malformations (risk ratio, 2.71; 95 percent confidence interval, 1.72 to 4.27) as compared with infants who had no exposure to antihypertensive medications. In contrast, fetal exposure to other antihypertensive medications during only the first trimester did not confer an increased risk (risk ratio, 0.66; 95 percent confidence interval, 0.25 to 1.75). Infants exposed to ACE

Hypertension and Kidney Disease

inhibitors were at increased risk for malformations of the cardiovascular system (risk ratio, 3.72; 95 percent confidence interval, 1.89 to 7.30) and the central nervous system (risk ratio, 4.39; 95 percent confidence interval, 1.37 to 14.02)."

The cardiovascular system abnormalities in this study included **atrial septal defect** (a hole between the top halves of the heart), **patent ductus arteriosus** (a normal connection from the artery to the lung to the main artery to body which typically closes at birth), ventricular septal defect (a hole between the bottom halves of the heart), and pulmonic stenosis (a narrowing of the pulmonary heart valve or main pulmonary artery). The nervous system defects included **hydrocephalus** (extra fluid in the brain areas), microcephaly (small brain), spina bifida (failure of the vertebrae in the spinal column to close), and encephalocele (a kind of blister in brain tissue).

Before you panic and decide you'll never have children, a little reality testing is needed. While there were birth defects to be sure, let's use an example from this very study to illustrate some commonsense findings. Among the 209 mothers who took an ACE inhibitor during the first part of pregnancy, nine babies were born with cardiovascular defects amounting to less than 3 percent. Comparing that to 29,000 babies born to mothers who did not take an ACE inhibitor during the first part of pregnancy, the same cardiovascular defects were present in just a little less than 1 percent. This raises the common problem of the relative versus the absolute. Relatively speaking, there were three times as many birth defects in moms who took the ace inhibitor. Absolutely speaking, the difference was 2 percent in the babies affected. We suggest that the conclusion from studies such as this one is that caution must always be exercised in treating medical diseases in pregnant women.

The most important thing in addressing this question is to recognize the risks involved in going forward with the pregnancy when someone has hypertension and/or reduced kidney

Atrial septal defect

Congenital cardiac malformation of the atrium with a defect between the right and left sides of the atrium.

Patent ductus arteriosus (PDA)

A congenital heart defect wherein a child's ductus arteriosus fails to close after birth. Symptoms include shortness of breath and cardiac arrhythmia, and may progress to congestive heart failure if left uncorrected.

Hydrocephalus

A usually congenital condition in which an abnormal accumulation of fluid in the cerebral ventricles causes enlargement of the skull and compression of the brain, destroying much of the neural tissue.

function. The best advice we know to give is for the pregnant woman to be under the care of an experienced team who recognizes these risks.

28. My doctor was concerned that my kidney arteries are blocked. Why would she think that?

First off, let's name this. When kidney arteries are blocked, we call that **renal artery stenosis**. "Renal" refers to the kidney, artery is pretty straightforward, and "stenosis" means narrowed or blocked. We suspect renal artery stenosis is present when we find blood pressure that is difficult to control, particularly in someone whose kidney function is reduced. Many times cigarette use over many years contributes to this kind of narrowing in the kidney artery. Clinically, we sometimes see significant changes in kidney function that are related to specific medications such as ACE inhibitors and angiotensin receptor blockers. These changes are more than the acceptable reductions that we discussed in Question 25. Another circumstance where we suspect renal artery stenosis is when a patient presents with heart failure, yet appears to have good heart function. In that situation, the heart failure seems to arise not because the heart itself is damaged but because the kidneys are unable to excrete the daily salt load effectively. This causes a backup in salt water in the body and leads to the pulmonary congestion we call heart failure. If the kidney arteries were not so blocked, it would not have happened.

Renal artery stenosis

Narrowing of one or both the renal arteries.

There are some clues to physical examination that also lead us to wonder whether renal artery stenosis is present. Sometimes we hear noises over the kidney arteries themselves, which are called bruits. Similar to a heart murmur, bruits are related to the turbulence of the blood flowing in the circuit. When the kidney arteries are narrowed, it creates a turbulent blood flow that we can sometimes hear with a stethoscope. We also suspect the kidney arteries may be narrowed when we see or hear evidence of narrowing in other arteries such as the carotid arteries in the neck, or the coronary arteries, because of a prior heart attack or from the results of a heart catheterization.

In summary, the things that make us think about renal artery stenosis are drug-resistant hypertension, in a smoker, with a bit of reduced kidney function, particularly if we are able to hear turbulence in the kidney arteries or know of narrowing in other blood vessels. The story does not stop there.

There is another kind of kidney artery narrowing that is not due to typical hardening of the arteries. This type of renal artery stenosis is due to abnormalities in the vessel that are related to the muscle layer of the vessel, not the lining. It's usually the lining that's affected in a hardening of the arteries, like that which is commonly called atherosclerosis. The renal artery stenosis related to the muscle layer is usually called **fibromuscular dysplasia**, or FMD for short. It's more common in women and typically shows up at a younger age. Renal artery stenosis like that described in the first part of this answer is typically a disease of the 65-year-old. FMD on the other hand typically shows up in a 40-year-old woman. In both cases, the elevation of blood pressure seems to be related to the narrowing of the kidney artery itself. As physicians, we are usually able to differentiate FMD from atherosclerosis-related renal artery stenosis based on the history and the patient's age. Ultimately, it depends on how the artery appears to the radiologist's eye in a test like an arteriogram.

Fibromuscular dysplasia

Abnormal proliferation of the muscular component of the artery resulting in narrowing of the renal artery lumen.

29. My blood pressure has been very difficult to control. If my blood pressure remains high, will this affect my kidney function?

The answer here is a very definite "probably." Most doctors know patients whose blood pressure goes on year after year badly controlled (for any of a dozen different reasons) with no visible consequence. Winston Churchill, for example, enjoyed an occasional alcoholic beverage, a good cigar, and had high blood pressure for many years during an era when there was no blood pressure therapy. He survived to a ripe old age. Most people whose blood pressure remains high get into some kind of trouble ultimately. The two biggest consequences of prolonged elevations in blood pressure are heart failure and stroke. In 1955, Dr. George Perrera, from Columbia University, published a large study of the natural history of untreated high blood pressure. Dr. Perrera related the stories of 500 patients who had high blood pressure that typically began in their 30s. All the patients died in his study, most about 20 years after diagnosis. His study addressed the answer to this question and showed that somewhere around 6 percent of the patients died from kidney complications due to uncontrolled high blood pressure. If you look carefully at his data, the number of people with impaired kidney function (which we have said previously contributes to cardiovascular disease) was closer to 20 percent.

The answer to this question is "probably." After practicing medicine for more than 20 years, words like "always" and "never" tend to disappear from your vocabulary. Medicine can be quite humbling—especially when you think you finally understand something and the next patient you see turns your well-understood knowledge base completely on its head.

You might wonder, then, why we treat everyone? The simple answer is that there's no way to identify ahead of time the one Winston Churchill from those who are not so gifted with the ability to survive, despite habits and vital signs that we know are not conducive to longevity. In the end, medical therapies such as treating high blood pressure are a trade-off of the benefits likely to accrue to a patient versus the risks of that therapy. In general, the risks of blood pressure treatment are relatively low, and the risks from uncontrolled high blood pressure are reasonably high. As a result we usually err on the side of treatment.

30. Is not using salt as important when I have both kidney disease and high blood pressure?

Restricting one's salt intake when both kidney disease and high blood pressure are present is even more important than when either is present alone. You could think of salt as gasoline and the interaction of kidney disease and high blood pressure like a bonfire.

What happens when you toss gasoline onto a bonfire? (Please don't try this one at home!)

If you reduce your salt intake, you reduce the likelihood that your blood pressure will need to rise in order to promote the excretion of the salt you consume in your diet. There is a finding in medicine called "salt sensitive hypertension." This means that some people have clear increases in their blood pressure when they eat salt. Not everyone dies, and some groups of people are more likely compared to other groups of people to have such increases when they consume salt. Let's take some examples.

Patients of African-American descent are more likely to have salt sensitive hypertension. Patients who are older, who are overweight, or who have kidney disease are all more likely to have salt sensitive hypertension. If you are a 65-year-old African-American with reduced kidney function and have a little trouble seeing your toes when you stand up, you are really likely to have salt raise your blood pressure further when you commit those occasional indiscretions such as visitations to fast food restaurants.

Diuretic

Substance or medication that causes an increase in urine excretion.

Even with good **diuretic** treatment, and diuretics are one way to promote the loss of salt from the body without resorting to elevated blood pressures, restricting salt intake makes the diuretic treatment even more effective. Finally (and there may be enough arrows sticking in this one already), higher salt intakes increase the amount of urinary protein loss. You'll recall that losing more protein in the urine is not a good thing. For all the above reasons, it's a great idea to practice abstinence when it comes to salt use. Can we hear an Amen please?

David's comments:

Initially, when consulting a nephrologist, the swelling in my ankles was brought to my attention. They were nearly twice the size they should be. The recipe was kidney disease + high blood pressure + a diet rich in salt. Now, by paying attention to the sodium content on food labeling and hidden salt content in most foods, I can see a dramatic difference in my ankle size. They are still a bit swollen but overall they are much, much better.

31. My blood pressure is pretty good right now, but my doctor wanted to add an extra medication anyway because of a finding in my urine test. What could make her think that way?

The most likely thing that would make your doctor think this way is the finding of persistent proteinuria, even with good blood pressure control. Picture two patients; both patients have the same blood pressure, in this case 128/74 mm Hg. Both have an eGFR of 45 mL/min/1.73m². They're both 50-year-old, African-American women. One has a negative-dipstick when protein was checked in the urine (this is good; negative is the medically correct result to have when a dipstick is placed in a urine sample). The other one has a dipstick that reads "++" (pronounced "two plus") when the urine is checked for protein. This is often pursued further by measuring the actual concentration of albumin (or protein) and creatinine in the urine. We'll talk more about that later. What will happen to these two women over time?

Our current knowledge suggests that the woman who has the detectable proteinuria will have more rapid loss of kidney function over time compared to the woman who does not. When we have intervened in clinical trials with drugs that both lower the blood pressure and lower the urinary protein loss, one of the most important things we have learned is that when the urine protein is reduced, it's as useful as the reduced blood pressure in preserving kidney function in the long haul. Consequently, one of the ways in which we aim to maximize what's left of kidney function is to use drugs specifically to reduce the urine protein loss further—even if we have good blood pressure control currently. There is no absolute number, or absolute dipstick finding that drives this decision. It's made on a patient by patient or case by case basis. There are other things that are factored into the decision to treat someone with additional medication for the specific purpose of lowering their urinary protein losses further since there are potentially some risks with these treatments. The biggest risk at this level of eGFR is an increase in the serum potassium concentration. The risk is small, on the range of a few percent. That's not very comforting when you're one of the "few percent" and experience the side effect.

One lesson the authors have learned reinforces a saying popular in Texas years ago. The saying goes like this: "When your horse is dead, it's time to get off." The lesson here is that when we do add medication, and check for the benefit (in this case reduced urine protein excretion) and don't find the benefit, we stop the medication. Those of you with kidney disease know well that you feel like you are single-handedly putting your pharmacist's kids through college, and treating physicians really do try to be sensitive to the number of pills we ask you to take. Honest.

32. I am on an (ACEI) ace inhibitor (lisinopril) and my doctor said type 2 diabetics should be on a different type of medication called an ARB (angiotensin receptor blocker). Is this true?

We hope as physicians that we make choices about how to treat patients based upon good evidence of benefit. We don't want to sound like a broken record, but it's important to preface this answer with that reminder. The answer to this question has to be formulated with some background first. Here goes the background.

We think that you are a type 2 diabetic who has some reduction in kidney function. Two very large trials of patients with diabetes and reduced kidney function demonstrated less loss of kidney function over time when the patients were treated with an ARB compared to identical blood pressure reduction using blood pressure medicines that did not include an ARB. So why don't I just say yes and go onto the next question? Glad you asked!

Neither of these two large studies compared an ARB to an ACE inhibitor. Consequently, the answer "yes" to the question is technically true because ARBs have been used in large trials and shown the benefits on what are called hard outcomes such as death, the need for dialysis or a transplant, and the worsening of kidney function reflected in a doubling of the creatinine concentration in the blood.

When a medicine is used to treat a medical condition, we call that condition an indication. If a patient has strep throat proven by culture, we know that penicllin is a drug used for this indication according to the FDA. For a type 2 diabetic with protein in the urine, two ARBs (losartan and irbesartan) are indicated for the treatment of diabetes and these changes in the urine, which we call nephropathy. For a type 1 diabetic with protein in the urine, the ACE inhibitor captopril is indicated. In both type 2 and type 1 diabetes, the treatment is indicated to preserve kidney function over time. All sorts of problems and confusion have arisen over years that have followed these clinical trials. For example, if two different ARBs worked well will all ARBs work? Since ARBs and ACE inhibitors are relatively similar in their blood pressure lowering and urine protein excretion lowering effects, it would seem that they would work pretty much the same way on everyone. At this time, we just don't know if that's true.

The United States Renal Data System publishes a report each year on the causes of kidney failure that lead to the need for dialysis or kidney transplant.

Based on the evidence, we would agree with your doctor. Whether you should switch medications, especially if you're well controlled at this point and have minimal or no urine protein loss, cannot be answered in a format like this book. There are sometimes other considerations present that lead a treating physician to use one medication versus another. Moreover, new data available this year (2008) from a large study called ON-TARGET, which compared an ARB to an ACE inhibitor. Technically speaking, it's not a kidney study, but there is information about this aspect in the study. The results showed ARB and ACE inhibitors to be equivalent when used alone. There was no advantage in combining these two drugs for cardiovascular disease protection.

33. My doctor said my severe high blood pressure caused my kidney disease and that I had primary hyperaldosteronism or Conn's syndrome. Is this true?

It could be. We mentioned previously that the kidney can be both victim and villain with high blood pressure. The United States Renal Data System publishes a report each year on the causes of kidney failure that lead to the need for **dialysis** or **kidney transplant**. Diabetes is number one and high blood pressure is number two on the list of causes. Consequently, the first part of this question indicating that high blood pressure caused your kidney disease is well based in fact. The second part of your question could be that both are true and related, or both true but unrelated. So let us explain that doubletalk a bit further.

Primary hyperaldosteronism or Conn's syndrome is a disorder where the **adrenal glands** make too much of a hormone called aldosterone. If you were to write up the job description for aldosterone, it would be pretty simple. Its job is to retain sodium at the expense of potassium. It's a great hormone to have if you're undertaking a trek across the Mojave Desert but forgot to take along some salt tablets. As you sweat and

Dialysis

A medical procedure to remove wastes or toxins from the blood and adjust fluid and electrolyte imbalances in patients with kidney failure or end stage renal disease.

Kidney transplant

A procedure in which a patient with severe kidney failure receives a kidney transplant either from a cadaver or deceased donor or a living donor who is often a relative or spouse.

lose salt through the skin, aldosterone comes to your rescue and after a few hours your sweat becomes virtually salt free. However, when the adrenal glands release aldosterone without such a stimulus like weather extremes, the effect is not so salutary. You would retain salt when you don't need to which raises blood pressure and causes some potassium loss in the process. The way in which they could both be true and related is that the high blood pressure of unrecognized aldosterone excess is often very difficult to treat. When you recognize aldosterone is present in excess there is a very specific remedy for it. Whether it's unrecognized aldosterone excess or just plain old difficult to control high blood pressure doesn't matter. Both can damage the kidney from the prolonged exposure to the elevated pressure.

Moreover, recent aldosterone research suggests one additional feature that is important and potentially related to this question. When aldosterone in excess is given to an animal, and it develops high blood pressure as a result, it also develops inflammation in target organs like the heart. Thus, it may be that the years of aldosterone exposure have not only driven up the blood pressure and contributed to reduced kidney function by that means, there may also be some scarring in the kidney as a result of the aldosterone excess.

Primary hyperaldosteronism:

Autonomous secretion of the hormone aldosterone either due to a unilateral benign adrenal tumor (or adenoma) or due to bilateral adrenal hyperplasia due to overproduction of aldosterone by both adrenal glands.

Adrenal glands

The two small endocrine glands located just above the kidneys. The adrenal glands secrete sex hormones, cortisol, and adrenaline (epinephrine).

Hypertension and Kidney Disease

PART FOUR

Diabetes and Kidney Disease

Should my blood pressure be controlled differently
if I have diabetes?

Does my sugar control affect my diabetic
kidney disease?

What is the most important factor in preventing my
diabetic kidney disease from getting worse?

More . . .

34. My doctor says I have microalbuminuria. What does that mean?

While we have addressed microalbuminuria in previous questions, we haven't done so specifically with regard to diabetes. What does microalbuminuria mean in a diabetic?

It means a bit more than the average population. Microalbuminuria is considered a marker, or a red flag, for things that could adversely affect kidney function in the future. As a matter of fact, the American Diabetes Association recommends that physicians treating a diabetic check for the presence of microalbuminuria yearly. They make this recommendation because of the high risk of overt proteinuria occurring when microalbuminuria is present. Finding a small amount of albumin in the urine in a diabetic signals a high likelihood that in the future the amount of protein will become visible on a dipstick. When a positive dipstick finding occurs within three to five years kidney function starts to decline dramatically.

It isn't hopeless, however. You can treat the microalbuminuria. Both ARBs and ACE inhibitors have been employed to treat microalbuminuria. However, there are other considerations when the patient is a diabetic. In a diabetic, better blood sugar control will often improve the microalbuminuria. We've also mentioned salt intake and reinforcing the need to be cautious with salt intake can also help reduce microalbuminuria.

Successful reduction of microalbuminuria to normal levels of urine protein excretion can occur by the use of the measures outlined above. If you are a type 2 diabetic with microalbuminuria, Dr. Hans Parving's research studies published in the *New England Journal of Medicine* on September 20, 2001, suggest that your chances of reverting back to normal levels of urine albumin excretion over a two-year period with aggressive use of an angiotensin receptor blocker is about 34 percent.

35. Should my blood pressure be controlled differently if I have diabetes?

There are different answers to this question, depending on treatment goals and if there are complications due to the diabetes.

The treatment goal with regard to diabetes is different from uncomplicated high blood pressure because the treatment goals are lower. If you have uncomplicated high blood pressure, we usually aim for a blood pressure less than 140/90 mm Hg as our control goal. When diabetes is present, we reduce that goal to the more difficult to obtain level of 130/80 mm Hg. As you can imagine, or as you have experienced if you have diabetes, getting to this lower goal usually requires more medication, and often more dedication to the lifestyle measures such as salt restriction that help the medications get you there. This lower treatment goal is based on a number of studies showing that when you lower blood pressure even beyond the regular 140/90 mm Hg goal, you get additional benefit in preventing target organ damage in patients with diabetes. This has not been so true in people with uncomplicated high blood pressure. Uncomplicated, when it refers to high blood pressure, means that you've got blood pressure elevation; period. It means you don't have diabetes, known heart disease, a prior stroke (or the threat of one), or kidney disease. You could have high cholesterol, for example, but you would still be uncomplicated. Uncomplicated refers specifically to evidence that high blood pressure has not taken a toll on one of the precious target organs: the heart, the brain, the kidney, or the circulation in general.

It is also important to know if complications are present. The particular complication we look for when choosing blood pressure medication is the presence of protein in the urine. We've covered this in detail in previous questions so we won't dwell on it at length here but it does influence the answer to

Diabetes and Kidney Disease

the question. When there is specifically protein present and measurable in the urine, we tend to prefer using medications that not only lower blood pressure but also seem to address the urine protein losses better than other medications. At the time of this writing the ACE inhibitors and the angiotensin receptor blockers are drugs in this category and are frequently used in the management of hypertension in patients with diabetes.

One way we try to implicate the presence of diabetes as the cause of kidney disease is by pursuing the history of eye involvement due to diabetes.

36. How do I know if diabetes is the cause of my kidney disease?

If you have ever played the game Clue® you'll be equipped to approach the answer to this question. First there is the crime. In this case, reduced kidney function. Then there are the suspects. When there are highly suspicious characters present in the patient's history aside from the presence of diabetes, we suspect that diabetes is the cause of kidney disease.

Retinopathy

Pertaining to harmful effects in the back of the eye (i.e., the retina).

Laser surgery

Surgery that is performed with a specific type of laser to treat eye disease in diabetics or diabetic retinopathy.

Let us give an example. Diabetes often affects the blood vessels in the back of the eye. This is called **retinopathy**. Interestingly, diabetes affects the kidney blood vessels in a similar way. Just as there is leakage of protein in the eye, there is leakage of protein in the urine. One way we try to implicate the presence of diabetes as the cause of kidney disease is by pursuing the history of eye involvement due to diabetes. Patients with retinopathy have often been told that they have it by their eye doctors, and frequently have undergone things like **laser surgery** to treat it.

More evidence accumulates when the urine reflects the presence of protein. It is unusual for diabetes to affect the kidney and not cause proteinuria. It can happen, but it's pretty rare. This is one of those situations where we sometimes consider a kidney biopsy because the pattern we see clinically is not typical of diabetes-related kidney disease. Another circumstance that points us away from diabetes causing the kidney disease is the presence of hematuria which is discussed in Question 13. It's not impossible, it's just less likely. Most of the time diabetes does not result in hematuria.

A few other items factor into the relationship. With type 1 diabetes, we usually know when it began. The natural history of type 1 diabetes and its associated kidney disease typically has a lapse of about 15 years between the onset of the diabetes and the development of kidney disease. With type 2 diabetes, it's not so clear because the onset is not recognized for years in some patients. The kidney disease tends to occur somewhere between 10 and 20 years after the diagnosis of type 2 diabetes but the time line is not understood as well as type 1. Moreover, patients with type 2 diabetes are older than those with type 1. Not uncommonly, they weigh more and have other exposures such as cigarette use in their past, all of which can contribute to blood pressure increases.

Finally, you might wonder how common diabetes-related kidney disease is if you have diabetes. With type 1 diabetes the chances of someday having kidney disease are about one in three. With type 2 diabetes, it's more of an educated guess but it's likely to be in the same range.

David's comments:

On my initial visit to see a kidney specialist, I was told that diabetes was the probable cause of my kidney disease. There were tests done to eliminate the different options and in the end the culprit was just as the doctors figured. Diabetes. The explanation for the protein leakage in both the eyes and kidneys was right on and masterfully illustrated by Dr. Townsend and Dr. Cohen. Bravo!!!

37. Does my sugar control affect my diabetic kidney disease?

You would think after many years of recognizing the relationship between having diabetes and developing kidney disease that this answer would have a slam dunk two-liner. Get ready for some disappointing news here. The answer is "Possibly."

The medical research that has been undertaken to evaluate the consequences of good versus not-so-good blood sugar control in patients with diabetes has had a checkered history. What we can say is that the weight of evidence suggests that better blood sugar control reduces the complications of diabetes such as the retinopathy, the neuropathy, and probably the kidney disease (or nephropathy). We did mention in Question 11 that some non-blood-pressure issues influence microalbuminuria. To this list we could add blood sugar control. A logical question to ask at this point is: "Why don't we know more about this?" To perform the kind of study necessary to really address well the answer to this question would take many years, cost lots of money, and require many people with diabetes to participate, since you won't see the endpoint (kidney function loss) in all the patients.

This brings up a common principle that underlies diabetes management. Even if perfect blood sugar control did not prevent kidney disease in the vast majority of patients, good blood sugar control has other benefits on the eye and the nervous system and is worth pursuing for those reasons. In the meantime, our hope is that medical research will continue to provide answers to how we can optimally manage diabetes and, hopefully, prevent or delay all the complications. Such an approach to care requires a pretty large team of professionals. An example of one such team comes from the STENO study in Denmark. If you're interested in reading further, pop into a library that subscribes to the *New England Journal of Medicine*, ask them for the January 30, 2003, issue and look at pages 383–393. You won't need an M.D. after your name to get the point that aggressive management of known cardiovascular risk factors in patients with diabetes can make a big difference in heart disease and stroke. One of these factors is blood sugar control. Also note the fact that such attention to detail requires a physician, a dietitian, a clinical nurse educator, and a few other folks all working together for the same end.

38. What is the most important factor in preventing my diabetic kidney disease from getting worse?

The answer right now is actually a deadlock. Two factors are neck-in-neck in the race for the most important thing to prevent, or slow down the progression of, kidney disease in patients with diabetes. They are familiar terms to you by now, assuming you haven't been skipping questions up to this point. If you have been skipping, not to worry—the authors are heavily into repetition!

Who are these two partners in cardiovascular crime? Suspect A is the familiar elevated blood pressure, and suspect B is the presence of protein in the urine. If we sound like a broken record, or to put it in a more chronologically correct analogy, a CD stuck on repeating track three, it's for a good reason. Briefly, that reason is that less than one third of patients with diabetes and high blood pressure have good blood pressure control. It's even harder to come by the statistics on how well we're doing on managing proteinuria. From a medication standpoint, it's usually easier to lower the blood pressure to goal than it is to lower the urine protein losses to normal.

Our colleagues would also chime in at this point to remind us that patient adherence to the prescribed regimen is also a significant factor. The authors have the greatest of sympathy when managing a patient with diabetes and kidney disease, particularly when their blood cholesterol is high. We tell them to restrict starches for the sake of the blood sugar, we tell them to restrict their dietary fat intake for the sake of the cholesterol level, and we warn them against the dangers of high protein intake when kidney disease is present. When they ask us "What on earth can we eat?" we could respond with "Well, water is pretty low in all of the above." Such responses are rarely met with a chuckle. Of course we never do that, but it does make dietary manipulation on the part of the patient a substantial challenge. Because of that challenge, it is important to have a dietitian and nurse educator assist the patient.

David's comments:

Juggling the diet restrictions to find foods that are low in salt, low in fat, low in protein, low in potassium, trans fat free, low in cholesterol, low in calcium, and low in carb is the mission of a dietitian. Food labels are tricky, and there are plenty of hidden things, and then even if you have the correct foods, you have to know how to prepare them. So having a consultation with a dietitian is a key ingredient to the success of your quest in the battle of kidney disease. This is something we as patients have direct control of.

39. I have had laser eye treatments and my doctor said that eye involvement or retinopathy usually occurs in diabetic patients with kidney involvement. Is this true?

Yes, it's quite true. It's so true that we actually have a term for it; renal-retinal syndrome. This term was popularized by a clinical kidney doctor named Eli Friedman years ago. It emphasizes the common **pathogenesis** in these separate organs linked by the blood vessel disease and the presence of diabetes.

Pathogenesis

Pathogenesis is the mechanism by which a certain etiological factor causes disease (pathos = disease, genesis = development).

The authors have found it to be pretty uncommon for a patient with a history of laser surgery in the eye to have absolutely perfect kidney function. That, however, raises an interesting problem called "referral bias." This is where a disclaimer comes into play. The authors are both nephrologists, so we tend to see patients with kidney disease. If the patient didn't have kidney disease, they would be less likely to see us. This means that when patients have had retinal complications from diabetes requiring laser surgery, but have not been referred to a kidney doctor because their kidney function seems normal, we would be unaware of these folks. When we look carefully at the patients we see who have had laser surgery on the eye, the kidney disease–diabetes connection is pretty clear. We went to some lengths to discuss this here because it's not an uncommon problem in some of the sensational reports that appear in the medical literature from time to time. Such reports can occasionally create panic among patients who have the particular disease that's part of the news story. Witness, for example, the recent furor over over Avandia, a widely prescribed diabetes drug. When the information regarding Avandia and heart disease was evaluated by a cardiologist, a substantial relationship between taking Avandia and having heart disease was noted by the cardiologist. However, when the data are looked at by other people such as the FDA or the company that markets the drug, or when you talk to physician-in-the-street who prescribes the drug, the relationship has not been so clear. That's why the authors respond to patient inquiries about recent headlines with an attitude of "Yes there may be something important here, but often there's more to this story than we see right now. Are you having a problem right this minute?" If we can ascertain that the patient is the same this morning as he or she was yesterday morning, then we do our best to give it a little bit of time to allow cooler heads to prevail and the data to be looked at a little more before making treatment decisions in a patient who is not currently experiencing difficulty.

So returning to our question, after this lengthy aside, what do we do with a "yes" answer to it? We submit that the first thing is that armed with this knowledge, it makes it incumbent upon physicians to be sure that diabetics are referred to ophthalmologists for periodic eye examinations. Diabetic retinopathy is one of the most common causes of preventable blindness. It also drives research into better ways to manage the blood pressure, the blood sugar, and other risk factors to serve better the goal of preserving vision.

40. Is there any treatment that can prevent my kidneys from getting worse and eventually requiring dialysis?

On the surface, this may look very similar to Question 38 but there is a bit more dimension to this one and that's why we took it separately. The answer now requires a broader consideration of what can be done in a patient with diabetes to preserve his or her kidney function maximally and to avoid requiring dialysis or, by natural extension, a kidney transplant.

In prior questions we have emphasized the role of good blood pressure control, urine protein reduction, and adherence to the lifestyle measures recommended by doctors based on research and typically carried out with the help of dietitians and diabetes nurse educators. What else is there? Now is the time to become even more comprehensive in the answer to this question. It's not an inconsequential concern, because we currently spend more than $20 billion a year in managing dialysis and the medical care in the first few years following a kidney transplant. We spend somewhere around six percent of the Medicare budget on managing the final complications of progressive kidney disease when it comes to dialysis and kidney transplantation.

Cytokines

Any of several regulatory proteins, such as the interleukins and lymphokines, that are released by cells of the immune system and act as intercellular mediators in the generation of an immune response. Also called chemokine.

The list of possible things that could be done to prevent kidney function from getting worse is huge. There are many blood tests, for example, that measure things like inflammation and the potential to form scar in tissues like the kidney. We call them **cytokines** because they come from cells (thus the "cyto") and because they do stuff actively (thus the "kine"). Unfortunately, most of the stuff they do is bad. With limited research, we know that sometimes even when we use drugs like ACE inhibitors, we don't prevent kidney disease progression. This is true even though the drugs are used properly. Research shows that when cytokines behave, with the use of drugs like ACE inhibitors, more benefit is seen by the patient. When cytokines remain elevated, despite the use of a drug, patients tend to progress or progress more rapidly.

Next, we have 60 years of cardiovascular research courtesy of the Framingham Heart Study (which started in 1948) to build upon in addressing this question. Although we have only limited data to support this, we think that many things that cause heart disease to get worse are also likely to cause kidney disease to get worse. We are just beginning to see evidence that good cholesterol control, typically with the use of a class of drugs called "**statins**," can preserve kidney function. In the CRIC study we mentioned previously, we are examining the role of good cholesterol control in the progression of kidney disease and diabetes. It will take about two more years before we know. Cigarette use (and you'll note we have not been on that soapbox until now) is another factor that likely increases the rate at which kidney disease gets worse, with or without diabetes. For a lot of reasons, it is important to give up the habit if you're in the habit of enjoying the habit. Finally, one area that appears very important is body weight. The majority of people with type 2 diabetes who experience a loss of kidney function are overweight or obese. Although we're not sure exactly why, the extra weight seems to wear the kidneys out more quickly. It's possible this occurs through one of those nasty little cytokines we mentioned previously. The last 20 years has shown us that fat cells do far more than sit there and store fat. They make lots of trouble, by virtue of producing a variety of cytokines. As a result, it may very well be that attention to weight loss as a significant priority in the management of the patient with diabetes who has, or is at risk of, kidney disease will climb on the list of important factors and rival those which we covered in Question 38.

David's comments:

Medicare puts out a wonderful publication called "Medicare Coverage of Kidney Dialysis and Kidney Transplant Services." The booklet is full of helpful information. Get it free of charge by calling the Social Security Administration at 800-772-1213.

Statins

The statins (or HMG-CoA reductase inhibitors) form a class of hypolipidemic agents, used as pharmaceutical agents to lower cholesterol levels in people with or at risk of cardiovascular disease. They lower cholesterol by inhibiting the enzyme HMG-CoA reductase.

Diabetes and Kidney Disease

41. My insulin dose was recently decreased does this have anything to do with my kidney function?

It sure does, and it gives the authors a chance to extol further the virtues of what the kidneys do for us. Among these virtues is the metabolism of hormones like insulin. When the kidneys fail, their ability to metabolize insulin fails with them. You may not notice this much when you do not need insulin to control your blood sugar, or in recent times inhaled to control your blood sugar. However, if you take insulin regularly, when your kidneys fail it's frequently the case that the dose is adjusted downward, and in some cases insulin is actually discontinued. You might wonder how a person could stop insulin. Is there something about kidney disease that makes our native insulin less effective so that we need an insulin supplement sometimes?

Glad you asked that. The answer is "Yes—there sure is." When kidney disease declines, even in the absence of diabetes, a peculiar medical situation called "**insulin resistance**" is often present. This is one of those terms that is self-explanatory. It means that insulin doesn't work that well because the body is resisting its blood-sugar-lowering effect. What happens to a person with insulin resistance is that they make more insulin to try and overcome the resistance. This works for a little while, but as the resistance worsens and the need for more and more insulin builds up, eventually the pancreas (the source of insulin) becomes exhausted and says: "Enough already." When that happens, the pancreatic production of insulin no longer meets the body's need and the blood sugar begins to increase since it is no longer possible to make up for the insulin resistance with higher insulin production.

Insulin resistance is by no means limited to patients with kidney disease. Current estimates are that one adult in four in the United States has some degree of insulin resistance. The lesson in all of this is that people often have significant

Insulin resistance

A situation in which insulin has difficulty promoting sugar uptake into body cells (the cells are resistant). High levels of insulin and sometimes blood sugar result. People with insulin resistance are at higher risk for developing diabetes.

amounts of residual insulin production even when they are diabetic and are taking insulin shots or inhalations. When kidneys fail, even though insulin production by the pancreas may not have been good enough in the past, the lack of insulin being broken down by the kidneys as they fail now allows insulin to last longer. As a result, shots or other forms of insulin administration may be tapered or even discontinued.

42. My doctor prescribed neurontin for my neuropathy. Can I take this, and does the dose need to be adjusted?

Neurontin is one of many drugs that have been used safely in patients with chronic kidney disease and diabetes or other neurologic problems. Neurontin works by interfering with the GABA receptor. This receptor transmits some of sensations that we feel like pain, numbness, or tingling. Interfering with this receptor can sometimes suppress unpleasant neurologic sensations, such as those that occur in patients with diabetes. Often, the complaint by the patient is a numbness, tingling, or burning in areas that are covered by gloves and stockings; that is, the hands and feet. Patients with these problems are often quite distressed with the symptoms so it is reasonable to consider the use of drugs like Neurontin in managing this uncomfortable circumstance. We mentioned in Question 16 that it is sometimes necessary to alter the dosing of medications when they are specifically excreted by the kidney.

Interestingly enough, Neurontin is one of those drugs that does require dose reduction as kidney function declines. In patients with reasonably good kidney function, those with an eGFR of more than 60 mL/min/1.73m^2 (see questions 14 and 15) the dosage is unchanged from normal. In those with stage three kidney disease, the dosage is reduced by about one third to one half. For those with stage four kidney disease the dosage is about the same as stage three. In those with stage five kidney disease who were not on dialysis but have and eGFR of less than 15 mL/min/1.73m^2 the dose is about one fourth of normal. This kind of information is published in the Physicians' Desk Reference (or PDR for short) and also in the package insert that sometimes comes with your prescription. Unfortunately, as drugs become generic and lose their patent protection, this kind of information frequently disappears from the PDR, which is published yearly. In that case, it's necessary to research published research studies, old editions of the PDR, or, if you're physician's hospital is fortunate enough to provide this resource, from a drug information group within the hospital. Typically, the drug information group would be part of the hospital pharmacy program.

David's comments:

I suffer plenty of pain from neuropathy. The quality of life is pretty dismal from the leg pain. Then I was told about Neurontin. For me, it was a wonder drug. It's been about five years since I began the medication. I have been pain free since I began taking it. However, Neurontin is processed in the kidney. I was taking 1,800 mg daily. Dr Cohen cut the dosage back to 300 mg. I feared the horrid pain would return, but it didn't. Needless to say everyone is happy (happy being an understatement!).

43. My doctor said I should stop my metformin because my kidney function was getting worse. Metformin has been controlling my sugars well. Should I stop taking it?

This is an important clinical question, and one about which kidney doctors and endocrinologists sometimes differ. The issue has to do with the true magnitude of risk associated with metformin (whose trade name is Glucophage). In a nutshell, the risk is an unusual circumstance called "**lactic acidosis.**" Lactic acidosis can happen when severe infections are present in some patients or when their liver is so damaged that it cannot handle the usual lactic acid production. When metformin levels build up in the blood, they contribute to lactic acid build-up and lactic acidosis. The key issue is: "What

Lactic acidosis

Abnormal accumulation of increased lactic acid levels in the blood.

causes metformin to build up in the blood in the first place?" Part of the answer to this question has to do with the fact that metformin is metabolized and excreted by the kidney. Consequently, when kidney function is reduced, metformin can build up in the blood and could thereby contribute to this problem with lactic acidosis.

Let's take a moment and define this disorder further.

When the body uses glucose (the typical sugar of the body's metabolism) for energy, it metabolizes the glucose differently depending on the presence or absence of oxygen. In situations where oxygen is at a premium, such as in exercising muscle where the oxygen need greatly exceeds the oxygen delivery. Those of you who are typically couch potatoes on weekends, then decide one day to buy a pair of jogging shoes and see how quickly you can run the mile will recognize the clinical symptoms of this imbalance of oxygen need and oxygen de-livery when your leg muscles notify you of their dismay over this sudden change in your lifestyle! When oxygen availability is reduced relative to need, then glucose is used less efficiently as an energy source. One of the results of this kind of glucose use is the build-up of lactic acid. Fortunately, there is a backup system to handle this lactic acid load. The backup system is your liver. The liver metabolizes loads of lactic acid every day. Consequently, it has a huge reserve potential and so lactic acidosis is very unusual unless the production is huge or the liver is impaired. In certain circumstances, such as reduced kidney function, when metformin is used, the issue is one of production. What happens clinically is that the lactic acid begins to build up in the blood, causing extreme shortness of breath because that's how the body deals with acidosis. By breathing more often and deeply your body is trying to excrete the acid by converting it into carbon dioxide that your lungs can eliminate. The most important aspect of all this is that there is a risk of death when lactic acidosis is present and that's what the furor over metformin use when kidney function is impaired revolves around.

The reason for our original comment is that the opinion differs about this among kidney doctors is that lactic acidosis complicating metformin use is very unusual. Even if your kidney function does decline and you continue to take metformin, your chances of lactic acidosis are still relatively small. The problem is they're not zero and there is no way to predict who will have a problem.

Allow us to introduce another wrinkle into this issue. Those of you reading this book who have been scheduled to undergo (or have undergone) an X-ray using a dye called iodinated contrast media should recall that you were told to stop the metformin before the procedure and only restart if your creatinine is unchanged two days after you received the dye. The reason for this is that there is always the possibility of an acute decline in kidney function after the administration of X-ray dye, a situation that is known as contrast nephropathy. If you experience contrast nephropathy, your creatinine level goes up, which indicates that your kidney function went down. If you were taking a drug like metformin it would be likely to build up because of this loss in kidney function.

What to do if you are a diabetic on metformin or if you are taking metoformin for a different reason and have kidney function impairment? This is one situation where guidance is best sought from your prescribing physician rather than trying to get a feel for it from a book like this one. While we can tell you that the standard of care is that metformin's use should be curtailed when the serum creatinine is above 1.5 mg/dL in men and about 1.4 mg/dL in women and an X-ray with dye is performed. There are exceptions to this in clinical practice, made on a case-by-case basis. You should speak with your physician before making changes in your treatment regimen.

44. If I get a transplant, will the diabetic kidney disease recur?

This question is going to require a little bit of background before we give an answer. If you had diabetes in the first place, as the question would indicate, there is a risk it could recur in the years after a kidney transplant. If you did not have diabetes in the first place, you could still develop diabetes during the transplant period since some of the medicines used to prevent rejection have diabetes as an adverse reaction to the drug. Let's address that first part first.

Most patients with diabetes who undergo a kidney transplant will see diabetes recur in their transplanted kidney. If **islet cells** are transplanted at the same time, this may reduce the recurrence of diabetes in the kidney transplant. Changes in the transplanted kidney indicating diabetes is occurring again can be detected after about two years by a kidney biopsy; however, it usually takes years longer than this to see clinical evidence indicating diabetes is again at play in the transplanted kidney.

Islet cells

Cells in the pancreas that produce insulin.

We talked a bit about insulin resistance previously in question 41. Some of the transplant medicines, particularly the ones called methyl-prednisolone (prednisone) and the ones called **calcineurin inhibitors** can do this. The risks may be higher in some situations, such as a chronic hepatitis C viral infection that has contributed to the loss of kidney function. The other thing that happens in some patients after a kidney transplant is weight gain. Weight gain is a risk for developing diabetes which can, in turn, affect the transplanted kidney.

Calcineurin inhibitors

Specific type of medication that is given to suppress the immune system after receiving an organ transplant.

However, the potential for diabetes recurrence has never been viewed as a barrier to transplanting patients who have diabetes. The many years of kidney function available from a kidney transplant are thought to more than offset the downside of having diabetes recur in the transplanted kidney.

45. I was started on a new medicine called "Januvia" for my diabetes. Does the dose need to be adjusted for my kidney disease?

Januvia, or when called by its generic name sitagliptin, appeared in the United States market in 2006. Some people may be unaware of this drug so let's take a moment just to review what it does.

Januvia inhibits a protein called DPP-4. When this protein is inhibited, it facilitates a better insulin response to food ingestion and smoother blood sugar levels after a meal. Think of it like using oil on the squeaky wheel. Januvia is the oil. The net effect is that the overall blood sugar profile is lowered, and the adequacy of blood sugar control as measured by the HbA1C concentration looks better.

Once again, turning to the PDR, we find that this drug does require some dosage reduction when kidney function is impaired. In this particular case, the dosage is about half (50 mg instead of 100 mg daily) when the kidney function is between 30 and 50 percent of normal. The dosage is reduced to 25 mg when the kidney function is less than 30 percent of normal.

Using authors' license, we should say something at this point about how kidney function is defined when the PDR is used. Previously we defined an eGFR. The PDR, however, uses an older way to estimate kidney function which is known as the Cockcroft and Gault equation. Here's how it's calculated:

(140 – Age in years) × Weight in kg/72 × Serum creatinine level = Answer

Ready for a pop quiz? Try your hand at this one using the above formula. You are a man, 60 years old, who weighs 238 pounds and had a recent blood test showing that you're creatinine was 1.4. What would Cockcroft and Gault say about your kidney function? Let's plug in the data and see what pops out.

$(140 - 60 \text{ years}) \times 108 \text{ kg} / 72 \times 1.4 = \text{Answer}$

$80 \times 108/72 \times 1.4 = \text{Answer}$

$8640/100.8 = \text{Answer}$

$85.7 = \text{Answer (rounded up to 86)}$

Got a different answer? Did you convert the weight from pounds to kilograms by dividing by 2.2 (238/2.2 = about 108 kg)?

Let's assume you were pretty close and now you have an answer of 86. But 86 what? We need to fill in the units. In this case, the units are simply mL/min. There is no "1.73m²" attached to this value, as with the eGFR. The numbers mean pretty much the same thing. If we were to put this person into the kidney stage classification he would be stage two (see Table 2). For the purposes of answering this question, he would get the usual dose, 100 mg, according to current recommendations. If we switched around his **chromosomes**, substituting an X for his Y thus changing his gender to a woman, the same formula would apply. However, as we mentioned previously, women tend to make less creatinine so the way we correct the formula after arriving at the answer (in this case 86) would be to multiply by 0.85. This now reduces the answer to 73 mL/min (86 × 0.85 = 73). Still above 50, so the dosing is not changed.

Chromosomes

Thread-like strands that contain hundreds, or even thousands, of genes.

If you increase the creatinine to 2.5 mg/dL and redo it, the man would now be 48 mL/min and the woman 41 mL/min and both would be treated with less (the 50-mg dose daily instead of 100 mg daily).

PART FIVE

Other Causes of Kidney Disease

I have been taking Advil for months for arthritis. My doctor says this has caused my kidneys to fail. Should I stop taking Advil? What can I take for pain?

I was diagnosed with polycystic kidney disease. Does that mean I will develop kidney failure? Is there any treatment for polycystic kidney disease?

I was found to have a large number of cysts on my kidney ultrasound. What does this mean?

More . . .

NSAID

Non-steroidal
anti-inflammatory
drug. These drugs are
used for arthritis and
pain management;
examples include
ibuprofen, naproxen,
and aspirin.

*Any patient
with pre-
existing kidney
disease should
be cautious
about taking
NSAIDs
as these can
make kidney
failure worse
and sometimes
the changes
caused are not
reversible.*

**Interstitial
nephritis**

Inflammation of the
kidney usually due
to certain drugs such
as antibiotics and
sulpha-containing
drugs.

46. I have been taking Advil for months for arthritis. My doctor says this has caused my kidneys to fail. Should I stop taking Advil? What can I take for pain?

We call Advil a **non-steroidal anti-inflammatory drug (NSAID).** Other examples of NSAIDs are ibuprofen, Aleve, and naproxen sodium. NSAIDs can cause acute and chronic kidney disease or even kidney failure. Any patient with pre-existing kidney disease should be cautious about taking NSAIDs as these can make kidney failure worse and sometimes the changes caused are not reversible.

Now, let's look at these particular situations in some more detail.

"Acute kidney failure" means that kidney function abruptly declined. This is even more likely to occur when a patient takes NSAIDs and he or she is dehydrated. This happens because the NSAIDs constrict blood vessels, which decreases the blood supply to your kidney. This type of renal failure is usually reversible.

"Chronic kidney disease" is pretty much what it says with an emphasis on "chronic." Trying to define "chronic" is akin to trying to define beauty. You might get different answers depending on whom you ask. By and large, kidney doctors agreed that chronic usually means a change in kidney function that has persisted for longer than three months. In the case of NSAID usage, we think that they can cause chronic kidney disease through **interstitial nephritis**. The best way we know to explain interstitial nephritis is to say that it is very much like an allergic response in the kidneys. When such a response persists over time, the kidneys begin to accumulate scar tissue. Unfortunately, the scar tissue tends to replace normal kidney tissue. As you might expect, regular kidney tissue does a terrific job at clearing the blood of waste products, but scar is no substitute for the real McCoy. So when scar accumulates at the expense of regular tissue, well, you won't need a calculator for this one. The loss of regular tissue takes its toll on kidney function. At this time, we lack magic wands to change scar tissue back into regular kidney tissue. Thus, the words of Ben Franklin (or should we say Poor Richard?) come to mind regarding the ounce of prevention. In this case, we suggest that prevention = NSAIDs taken with caution at the lowest dose in patients who have normal kidney function but should be avoided if possible altogether in patients with underlying kidney function problems or kidney failure.

47. I had an infection and was treated with antibiotics 10 days ago. My doctor says this may have caused kidney failure. Is there any treatment? Is it reversible?

This situation represents an example of what the media would call "friendly fire." In this case, the well-intentioned use of an **antibiotic** had an unfortunate consequence on kidney function. Some antibiotics appear to be more likely to do this than others. The good news is that it's usually temporary.

Antibiotic

Medications prescribed to treat infections.

Antibiotics like penicillin and cephalosporin are associated with interstitial nephritis, which is when the kidney has what appears to be an allergic reaction to a drug. Think about what happens in your nose if you have allergies or what happens to someone you know who unfortunately is a ragweed casualty. Terms like "stuffy nose" come to mind. The stuffy nose results from swelling in the membranes of the nose. This produces the familiar blocked nasal passageway voice. The same kind of swelling occurs in the kidney in the presence of interstitial nephritis. Like the nose, when similar swelling occurs in the kidney, which has a capsule around it that keeps its size from expanding, the soggy kidney tissue is trying to swell with no room to do so. Consequently, it gets pretty tight in there and blood has a hard time flowing through the crowded kidney swelling. With less blood flow, the result is acute kidney failure, because it's clearly very hard to clear the blood if you're not given the blood to clear in the first place.

The good news is that usually just stopping the drug alone will result in improvement of kidney failure. Most patients will have complete return of kidney function if the kidney failure is recognized early enough. Sometimes the kidney failure is very severe, and you might require a course of oral steroids to decrease the kidney's allergic reaction. Allergic interstitial nephritis can be diagnosed with urine tests. Usually, there will be an increase in white blood cells in the urine and these white blood cells can cause casts, which a kidney specialist can identify by looking at your urine under a microscope. Once you have had acute interstitial nephritis, you should think twice before you take that particular drug again as this allergic reaction is likely to recur. Actually, you, your doctor, your pastor, and/or your rabbi, and/or other religious/social authority should probably all agree that the risks here outweigh the benefits before you undergo another go at your kidney function in the name of treating the latest microbial invader.

48. I have kidney disease and was told to avoid getting dye with a CT scan or MRI. Why is that? What if a test is absolutely necessary? Is there anything I can do to prevent getting kidney failure?

There is an old saying that goes like this: "You can't be a *little bit* pregnant." With pregnancy, it's all or nothing. Not so with kidney disease. The magnitude of kidney function impairment is an important part of answering this question. You can have just a *little bit* of kidney impairment. We'll get to that in a second, after we talk a little bit about what's involved in these two tests.

A CT scan or an MRI will often be administered with an intravenous dye that is injected into a vein in your arm. The dye used with a CT scan contains iodine and the dye used with an MRI is called **gadolinium**. People may be allergic to dye (or the "iodine contrast" as it's also called) if they have a seafood allergy which involves shellfish, like shrimp. Let's put this into some kind of perspective now. Less than 1 percent of people who receive iodine contrast will develop acute kidney failure if they have normal kidney function. People are more likely to develop kidney failure after exposure to contrast if they have abnormal kidney function. The particular level of kidney function that worries us is in stage 3. Moreover, the type of kidney disease matters also. For example, diabetics with kidney disease are even more prone to develop kidney failure (or worse kidney failure) when they undergo a CT scan that uses dye given by injection.

Gadolinium

Contrast agent or dye injected with MRI.

This brings up an important point. You may hear the radiology technician tell you about the contrast in your CT study. There are actually two kinds of contrast used. We have been going on about the one that is injected by vein, but there is also the kind that is swallowed so that your stomach and intestines can be identified in the X-rays. This swallowed contrast, or dye, stays in the intestines and does not molest your kidneys.

If you are undergoing a CT with contrast the usual advice is to be well hydrated prior to the scan and avoid using drugs such as Advil for a few days prior to the scan. There are a few other drugs such as ACE inhibitors like enalapril that might reduce blood flow to the kidney and predispose you to developing acute kidney failure. If the test is absolutely necessary and you have underlying kidney failure, you should ideally receive fluids such as normal saline through your vein for a day prior to the procedure. You could also take a medication called Mucomyst®. It's generic name is acetylcysteine and it may further decrease your chances of developing kidney complications from the dye. This situation calls for a huddle with your doctor(s) to figure out the best approach to preserve your kidney function during and after your scan. Once again, the good news is that acute kidney failure only occurs in 5–10 percent of high risk patients. It almost always occurs within 24–48 hours after receiving the IV dye load. As kidney doctors, we usually check the kidney function one to two days after the procedure. We think that if your creatinine is stable at 48 hours post-scan you will have avoided this complication. Okay, that's one scan down and one to go.

When a person is scheduled for an MRI scan it's a different situation altogether. This time the nasty stuff given by vein is gadolinium. It sounds like an aluminum company product, doesn't it? Gadolinium is a substance that has a particularly useful response when exposed to the strong magnetic field in an MRI. It highlights the blood vessel and gives the picture both of blood flowing to a tissue, and whether the tissue seems to enhance after the gadolinium is injected. Up until about 2003, we gave gadolinium without a second thought to patients with impaired kidney function and even on dialysis because we felt that the gadolinium was not toxic to the kidneys. Although we still doubt it's toxic to the kidneys, there are other tissues in the body besides the kidney. Nephrologists have often suspected that is a rumor. What we have learned recently is that gadolinium is associated with a particularly debilitating illness called **nephrogenic systemic fibrosis (NSF).** The occurrence of this complication is more likely in patients whose kidney function is reduced to 30 percent function or lower (stages 4 & 5). In these patients gadolinium should be avoided if at all possible. NSF causes severe thickening of the skin with stiffening of the joints and there is no current therapy that results in reversal of symptoms. When we absolutely have to do the MRI, we sometimes resort to **hemodialysis** right after the MRI with gadolinium injection is completed. Once again, this is the sort of thing that is best served by conferring with your health care provider(s).

Nephrogenic systemic fibrosis

A rare and serious syndrome that involves fibrosis of skin, joints, eyes, and internal organs. Its cause is not fully understood, but it seems to be associated with exposure to gadolinium. It does not have a genetic basis.

Hemodialysis

Dialysis of the blood to remove toxic substances or metabolic wastes from the bloodstream; used in the case of kidney failure.

49. I was found to have a large number of cysts on my kidney ultrasound. What does this mean?

Cysts can mean several things. They occur in the kidney as part of the normal aging process. If you are over the age of 35, odds are about one in three that you have at least one of these puppies in your kidneys. They don't usually produce symptoms so you wouldn't know unless you had an ultrasound done. Cysts come in several varieties. The main varieties are: simple and complicated. If the cysts are simple this means they are fluid filled without septations, which partition the cyst into compartments. Simple cysts are almost always benign and do not need any follow up. As you have probably guessed, the presence of septations in the cyst or cysts, or a funky appearance to the fluid itself inside the cyst, moves them into the category of complex or complicated. These are the guys that we usually pursue with further testing.

So, when a cyst is pretty big (for example, larger than 3 cm or about and inch and quarter) or appears to have a complex appearance on ultrasound, we consider a CT scan or an MRI to further determine if something like kidney cancer is present. Somewhere along the line, we dropped the ball about the "large number." Without further ado let's pick that ball up again.

We are going to need a little help from Mr. Webster's dictionary. We're going to introduce two new terms that are familiar, but which have specific meaning in "The Case of The Cystic Kidney." The first term is "multiple," and the second term is "polycystic." Multiple cysts can occur in one or both kidneys, but do not usually result in kidney enlargement and are not thought to be particularly ominous for future kidney function. Polycystic kidneys, on the other hand, also have multiple cysts, almost always in both kidneys, and almost always have enlargement of the kidneys on the ultrasound. Strangely enough this situation is called "polycystic kidney disease" (or PCKD). This is an inherited condition and is discussed further in the next question.

50. I was diagnosed with polycystic kidney disease. Does that mean I will develop kidney failure? Is there any treatment for polycystic kidney disease?

If you are one of those people that turns to the end of the story before reading the middle parts, but you have successfully resisted that temptation until now, the authors would like to grant you "reader's license" to go directly to the last question, do not pass go, do not collect a get-out-of-jail free card, or do anything else except to go directly to the last question for an example of how to use current Internet resources to pursue further knowledge about this condition. If you're one of those folks that would "never dream of doing that" (i.e., skipping ahead) then read on, and ignore the preceding sentence.

There are two types of PCKD that can affect the adult, and occur due to abnormal genes a person inherits on two different chromosomes. Occasionally a genetic mutation occurs spontaneously and there is no family history of cystic kidney disease. They are called type 1 and type 2.

Type 1 PCKD is more severe and you are more likely to lose your kidney function and progress to end stage kidney failure requiring either a transplant or dialysis. Type 2 PCKD is a milder form and often kidney failure only occurs very late in life or may not occur at all. The only way to definitively distinguish between these two types is to have genetic testing. That sounds easy, but it can be challenging because, since it is expensive and usually not covered by insurance, it is rarely done. If your relatives with PCKD developed renal failure in their 40–50s they likely have type 1 disease. If you have a relative with PCKD who only develops kidney failure in his or her 70–80s he or she are more likely to have type 2 disease, which is a milder form of the disease but may still lead to end stage kidney failure. Most patients initially present with high blood pressure long before their kidney function becomes abnormal. This type of kidney failure is not associated with protein leaking in the urine so conventional therapy aiming to reduce proteinuria, such as an ACE inhibitor or angiotensin receptor blocking drug, is not particularly helpful in preventing kidney failure in this type of kidney disease. However, lest the infant be cast away with the used bathwater, we hasten to say that it is still very important to control blood pressure well. Most patients will require several blood pressure drugs to control their blood pressure to a target blood pressure of 130/80 mm Hg or less. There is no proven treatment for PCKD to preserve kidney function at this time; however, research is being done on some promising treatments. One current drug trial is with a drug called tolvaptin. The theory is that tolvaptin causes less fluid accumulation in the cysts and slows progression of the disease. Tolvaptin has shown promising results in early trials and currently there is a large worldwide trial being conducted. There is also current testing looking at the volume of the cysts on a MRI to try to predict if a patient's renal function will deteriorate depending on the volume of the kidney cysts.

Most patients initially present with high blood pressure long before their kidney function becomes abnormal.

51. Will my children inherit this disease (PCKD)?

Odds are that you already know the answer to this question. We all know that some things just "run in families." Unfortunately, PCKD is one of those things that does, indeed, run in families. If you or the child's other parent has PCKD there is a roughly 50:50 chance for each child to also carry the PCKD gene. This doesn't mean that if you have four children, two will have PCKD and two will not. Unfortunately, genetics just doesn't work like that. You could have four completely unaffected children or four affected children. The main thing to keep in mind is that EACH child has the 50:50 chance of having the PCKD gene. So, how would you know?

Kidney cysts can occur early in childhood and an ultrasound is recommended in the late teens if one of the parents is affected. In order to make the diagnosis, a patient must have more than three cysts. If you have not developed any cysts by age 30, you can be pretty sure you (or your child) has not inherited the disease. Genetic testing is an option, but is very expensive and rarely done for that reason. Renal ultrasound is cheap and fairly easy to perform and is an excellent test to pick up cysts in the kidney, so usually no further testing is required.

52. If I require a transplant will the PCKD recur?

This is a great question. Recurrence of the primary kidney disease in the newly transplanted kidney is a frequently asked question. Because kidney transplants have been done for more than 40 years, we are actually getting pretty good at understanding what does or does not recur in the transplanted kidney.

PCKD does *not* recur in the transplanted kidney. Patients with PCKD usually do very well when they get a transplant, as they usually do not have other major medical issues. The patient may occasionally require surgery to have both kidneys they were born with removed prior to renal transplant if the kidneys are really large and are occupying a large amount of space in the abdomen.

53. I was diagnosed with "lupus nephritis." What does this mean?

On our first day of medical school, the authors were told that by the time they finished medical training they would have about 50,000 new terms to stuff in their already feverish minds. We have both found this to be woefully untrue. It's more like twice that. Consequently, we are extremely sympathetic when patients come to us using medical terminology, often with several web-based printouts, and begin the Q & A with a question like this one. Let's take the two terms apart and, using the advice that the Good Witch of the East gave to Dorothy in *The Wizard of Oz*, let's start at the beginning.

Lupus is derived from Latin, and means "wolf." There are two schools of thought as to how this term came to be associated with the disease that we call lupus. Since lupus often presents with a facial rash around the nose, it was thought that perhaps it resembled a wolf bite to the face. The other thinking had to do with how lupus can "devour" an affected organ. If you own a dog (a close cousin of the wolf) and have watched it eat, well—you have had a ringside seat to appreciate what "devour" really means.

Nephritis leverages two terms. The first-term is "nephro" from the Greek which refers to the kidney. The second part is the "itis," which refers to inflammation. I bet you see where this is going. Nephritis refers to an irritation or an inflammation in the kidney. This is usually manifested by things like blood or protein in the urine as we reviewed earlier in the second section of this book.

Don't think that lupus nephritis refers to a wolf with ailing kidneys. It refers to a patient who has lupus, which has now affected his or her kidneys in some way. Other organ systems are usually involved and most commonly include the skin and bone marrow. Most patients who are diagnosed with lupus nephritis will need a kidney biopsy to determine how severe the kidney involvement is. Treatment will depend on how severe the kidney disease is. Lupus is more common in females and African Americans and is more severe in African Americans. There is often a family history of lupus. Lupus nephritis is classified according to the pattern that is seen on the kidney biopsy. The various types of kidney involvement include:

- type 1 or normal kidney tissue

- type 2 or mesangial **glomerulonephritis**

- type 3 or focal proliferative glomerulonephritis (FPGN)

Glomerulo-nephritis

Inflammation of the glomeruli of the kidney; characterized by decreased production of urine and by the presence of blood and protein in the urine and by edema.

- type 4 or diffuse proliferative glomerulonephritis (DPGN)

- type 5 or membranous glomerulonephritis.

Type 2 and type 5 have the best prognosis but can occasionally get worse. Type 3 and 4 have the worst prognosis. Type 3 often progresses to type 4 and the patient diagnosed with type 3 or 4 will often develop end stage kidney disease and require dialysis or a kidney transplant. Patients usually have protein in the urine and the creatinine level may be elevated. The doctor will also order tests of the immune system including antineutrophil cytoplasmic antibody (ANA), which will be increased in lupus. The double-stranded **DNA** antibody blood test (DS DNA) will also be positive when a patient has kidney involvement due to lupus. **Complement levels** (C3 and C4) will also be checked and these are expected to be below normal when the lupus nephritis is active.

54. My doctor said I should get chemotherapy with cytoxan and steroids to prevent renal failure from lupus. Should I proceed with this treatment?

Some words have very scary connotations. For the authors, the word "**chemotherapy**" is certainly in that category. Normally, we associate this with some kind of drug treatment for cancer. Even if we hear it outside of the cancer context, our minds are drawn to the idea that this is life-and-death stuff. Let's first deal with the issue of what the word "chemotherapy" means. Once again we can dismiss the rocket scientist and simply look at the word. Here we have a compound word with two parts. The first part is chemo, meaning "drug" or "medication." The second part is therapy. We'll spare you hitting you on the head with this one. Now we have, hopefully, dealt with the anxiety associated with the use of this word. Let's go on then and discuss the essence of the question.

Treatment of lupus nephritis will depend on the pattern of kidney involvement that is seen on the kidney biopsy. Patients

---

DNA

A nucleic acid that carries the genetic information in the cell and is capable of self-replication and synthesis of RNA. DNA consists of two long chains of nucleotides, the sequence of nucleotides determines individual hereditary characteristics.

Complement levels

Proteins measured in the blood that are decreased in autoimmune diseases.

Chemotherapy

Form of medication that can be given orally or through a vein for cancer therapy and for some autoimmune diseases to suppress the immune system.

who have mesangial GN (glomerulonephritis) or membranous GN usually will not require low dose chemotherapy, and treatment will consist of ACE inhibitors or ARBS aiming to reduce urine protein and control blood pressure well to a goal of 130/80 mm Hg or less. If a patient has type 3 (FPGN) or type 4 (DPGN) lupus nephritis on the renal biopsy, these patients will usually require low dose chemotherapy to try to prevent kidney disease from getting worse. There are different treatment regimens, often with many side effects, so the treatment should be discussed in detail with the patient's kidney doctor. The reason for more aggressive treatment in type 3 and type 4 LN is because usually kidney function deteriorates fairly rapidly in these types of patients. Often they will go on to lose kidney function and require dialysis or a kidney transplant. Patients may require long term therapy and sometimes will be required to be treated a number of times. A patient may also need to have a repeat kidney biopsy to see if kidney disease is getting worse or if there is a lot of scar tissue and it is no longer worthwhile treating the kidney disease with such strong medications. Usual treatment consists of steroids in combination with Cytoxan or CellCept. All these therapies have serious side effects, and it is necessary to weigh up the benefits and risks of treatment.

55. If my kidneys fail due to the lupus will I be able to get a kidney transplant?

Yes.

That was easy, wasn't it?

It is usually recommended that patients wait a year after their disease has settled down before getting a transplant. Patients will usually require dialysis for a year before getting transplanted. Patients with lupus nephritis usually do well with a kidney transplant as the drugs given to stop the rejection of the new kidney will suppress the immune system and, in most cases, control the lupus. Recurrence rates after transplant with

It is usually recommended that a patient wait a year after their disease has settled down before getting a transplant.

lupus are about 1–4 percent. You are not completely out of the woods, but most of the trees will be behind you.

56. I had a cardiac catheterization and after the procedure my kidney function has slowly continued to get worse. Is this related to the catheterization procedure?

The authors have not been reticent to rush in where angels fear to tread when answering these questions. Although we recognize this response is likely to frost our cardiology companions, the answer is that cardiac catheterization can affect kidney function, and is more likely to do so if you have pre-existing kidney function impairment. Fortunately for all of us, however, cardiologists are well aware of this problem and take several precautions to reduce the likelihood. Let's pursue how the cardiac catheterization procedure might introduce things that could upset kidney function.

Cardiac catheterization can result in kidney failure in two ways. First, and most commonly, patients can experience acute kidney failure from the dye used in the cardiac catheterization. This is usually reversible, and patients at high risk (for example, diabetics with a creatinine of 3.0 mg/dL or higher) for this type of problem can be pretreated with intravenous fluids and a nasty smelling substance called Mucomyst® before the procedure.

Plaque

An area of hardening in the blood vessel.

Another way the heart catheterization procedure can cause kidney failure is through atheroembolic kidney failure. Atheroembolic kidney failure usually occurs after a catheterization when cholesterol **plaque** (that's where the "athero" part comes from) is disrupted. Tiny pieces of cholesterol are released into the blood and lodge in the kidneys and other organs like torpedoes (and this is where the "emboli" part comes from). This usually results in kidney failure that gets worse over a few weeks, rather than pretty much right away as with the dye administration in the first part of this answer. This can progress to end stage kidney disease with the patient requiring dialysis in some cases. Patients may also have these tiny cholesterol pieces, or emboli, embedded in other organs such as the eyes and the skin. If the back of the eye is examined by an eye specialist, they will be able to see **cholesterol emboli** called **Hollenhorst plaques** in the back of the eye. Patients may also have a lacy or fishnet-like pattern on their skin, particularly of the lower legs and around the knees. This is called livido reticularis (which translates basically into fishnet). Patients may also complain of loss of appetite due to involvement of the bowel vessels. Unfortunately, this type of kidney failure has a very poor prognosis and the kidney failure will progress. The patient will usually require dialysis a few weeks to months after the procedure. There is no way to prevent this from occurring. This type of renal failure occurs infrequently and is only present in 0.05 to 0.18 percent of all patients undergoing cardiac catheterization.

Cholesterol emboli

Small pieces of cholesterol that break off from a plaque and deposit in distant organs.

Hollenhorst Plaques

Cholesterol plaques seen in the retina or the back of the eyes due to deposition of atheroemboli or cholesterol emboli.

57. I have had repeated bladder infections. Can this affect my kidney function?

The answer to this one depends on how old you are when you pose the question. Repeated bladder infections in an adult usually do not cause renal failure; however, repeated urinary tract infections in infancy and childhood can be associated with reflux of urine repeatedly into the kidney. This can cause a type of chronic renal failure or worsening of kidney function over time. The best intervention is to treat the underlying cause of urinary tract infections in children. With repeated UTIs in childhood, a patient can develop reflux nephropathy, which eventually results in a scarring pattern in the kidney with progression of kidney failure to end stage kidney disease.

Keep in mind, though, that nothing is ever really simple. Question 47 discussed the use of antibiotics and how they affect kidney function.

MGUS

Abnormal accumulation of monoclonal proteins in the blood.

Clonal

Multiple identical copies of a DNA sequence.

Immunoglobulin

A protein produced by plasma cells which plays an essential role in the body's immune system. These proteins attach to foreign substances like bacteria and assist in destroying them.

Antibody

Proteins that are produced by the immune system in response to foreign substances called antigens. Each antibody is unique and defends the body against one specific type of antigen.

Gamma globulin

A type of protein found in the blood. When gammaglobulins are extracted from the blood of many people and combined, they can be used to prevent or treat infections.

58. I was diagnosed with abnormal proteins in my blood (MGUS). Can this affect my kidney function?

These proteins can sure make for a lot of trouble. One of the most fascinating things about the human genome project is that we have learned that there are at least 30,000 genes in the human DNA. That means that there are at least 30,000 gene products (which we usually call proteins) in the human. Imagine the size of the computer you would need in order to keep track of, for example, 30,000 bank accounts. It's amazing that it works so well so much of the time.

The difference between normal and abnormal can be quite subtle. In this particular case, the proteins are kind of screwed up. They are not the normal types of antibodies one would make if you were given a polio vaccine, for example. These proteins can either be shorter than usual, or far more abundant than usual. Either way, they make for trouble because they tend to build up and cause problems with kidney function. Let's expand the abbreviation **MGUS** and then finish up with an answer.

The letters MGUS stand for "monoclonal gammopathy of undetermined significance." Monoclonal becomes clear when you simply take it apart into its two terms. The first, mono, means one. The second term, **clonal**, refers to copies of something and is the source of our common vocabulary word clone. Putting it together, monoclonal refers to multiple copies of one thing. In this case the one thing is an **immunoglobulin** (sounds like a Halloween character doesn't it?), otherwise known as an **antibody**. Perhaps you've heard of someone who got a shot of **gamma globulin** after exposure to hepatitis. It's the same thing. Just imagine a gallon-sized syringe giving that gamma globulin and now you start to get the picture. Where does all that extra antibody go? If you answered "Perhaps to places like the kidney," you've hit the nail on the head. If the kidney gets soggy with all this extra gamma globulin it is harder for the kidney to do its job. This takes its toll and becomes evident in the blood and urine tests that doctors do to understand this problem. In the early stages an MGUS may be mild enough to not cause any trouble that would be picked up on the usual radar screens. The problem is an MGUS can transmute into something worse with time, something like **myeloma**, which is a cancer of **plasma cells** that produce antibody in the first place. That is the point at which problems with kidney function are usually noted.

59. I have myeloma and my doctor said I have abnormal kidney function. What could cause this? Will I need dialysis?

Myeloma can cause various types of kidney disease. The most common form of kidney involvement is cast nephropathy or myeloma kidney. This is due to a large amount of abnormal proteins in the blood being filtered by the kidney and blocking up the kidney tubules. A patient can get acute kidney failure, which may be reversible with treatment of the myeloma decreasing the amounts of these proteins in the blood and urine. Treatment consists of prednisone and chemotherapy (melphalan), and sometimes **plasmapheresis** (exchange of plasma) will be required. Patients may also require temporary dialysis if kidney function worsens. Often treatment will cause reversal of renal failure and dialysis is temporary. Some patients will also need a bone marrow transplant as a more definitive treatment for the myeloma. Myeloma can also cause chronic kidney disease that continues to worsen over a few months with complete loss of kidney function and need for chronic dialysis. Myeloma can result in very high calcium levels in the blood, which can cause dehydration and acute renal failure. This is usually reversible with fluids and lowering of calcium levels in the blood. High cell turnover due to cell breakdown from a tumor can cause high levels of **uric acid** and this can also cause ARF, which is also usually reversible. Patients with myeloma often need imaging studies with a CT scan and will receive intravenous dye and can develop contrast

Myeloma

A disseminated type of plasma cell dyscrasia characterized by multiple bone marrow tumor foci and secretion of an M component, manifested by skeletal destruction, pathologic fractures, bone pain, the presence of anomalous circulating immunoglobulins, Bence Jones proteinuria, and anemia.

Plasma cells

Cells of the immune system that secrete large amounts of antibodies.

Plasmapheresis

The removal, treatment, and return of (components of) blood plasma from blood circulation.

Uric acid

The end product of nitrogen metabolism. High levels of uric acid in the blood are associated with increased risk of uric acid kidney stones and gout.

Patients with chronic kidney failure due to myeloma generally do not have a good prognosis.

nephropathy due to the dye load. Other less common causes of renal failure include amyloid (abnormal proteins accumulate in the kidney and other organs causing chronic kidney failure), light chain deposition disease, and heavy chain deposition disease (abnormal proteins deposited in the kidney). Patients with chronic kidney failure due to myeloma generally do not have a good prognosis.

PART SIX

Treatment of Kidney Disease

I have been diagnosed with kidney disease. Is there any special diet I should follow?

I have chronic kidney disease. Can my kidneys get better?

Are there any medications I should avoid if I have kidney disease?

More . . .

60. I have been diagnosed with kidney disease. Is there any special diet I should follow?

What a great way to start an argument! Even between the two authors of this book there is some difference of opinion about this issue. One might wonder why we would have thought that diet might make a difference in the first place. Where did such a notion come from? The answer is buried in the period before dialysis became possible, yet at a time when kidney function could be measured accurately. This was in the 1940s and 1950s. It particularly came from the work of a doctor named Thomas Addis who recognized that one of the principal jobs of the kidney was to eliminate the waste products they came from eating protein in the diet. You might remember from your high school days about how proteins are built, not unlike Tinker toys, from basic units called **amino acids**. When amino acids are eaten in excess of the need to replace body proteins, they can be used for fuel just like **carbohydrates** and fats. The problem is dealing with the waste products. When the body "burns" carbohydrates and fats it generates carbon dioxide and water as the waste products. They are pretty easy to get rid of. When the body burns amino acids it also generates carbon dioxide and water BUT there is a twist to the story. The twist comes from the fact that carbohydrates and fats are made out principally of carbon, hydrogen and oxygen. So are amino acids with the interesting little twist that amino acids also have *nitrogen*. It's the nitrogen that causes the trouble since it has to be specially handled. That special handling produces a waste product called urea. If you are a gardening enthusiast you'll recognize that term immediately. When you buy a fertilizer and you see the three numbers on the outside of the bag, one of those three numbers refers to the urea content in the fertilizer. Urea is simply a combination of nitrogen and hydrogen sitting on either side of a single carbon atom. You might think such a simple molecule would be easy to get rid of, and it is, as long as your kidneys are functioning normally. When they're not functioning normally, and when the diet includes a generous

Amino acids

The smaller molecules that are joined to form proteins.

Carbohydrates

A common substance in foods that are broken down in the body to simple sugars and are a major source of energy for the body.

helping of protein, the resulting urea production causes work for the remaining kidney function to deal with. The logic here was "well, if we reduce the protein intake that will reduce the urea load and give the kidneys less work to do." Brilliant idea, but extremely difficult to achieve in practice, so it has remained somewhat controversial.

In general, it is still believed that if you reduce your dietary protein intake it may slow progression of kidney disease. However a large study (MDRD study) did not prove this to be true. There are many anecdotal experiences of slowing down the progression of kidney disease and most kidney doctors would recommend a moderately reduced protein intake in a patient with chronic kidney disease. A moderate intake would be 0.8 g of protein per kilogram of body weight per day. If one has a lot of protein in the urine then protein intake should be less restrictive and increased to 1 mg/kg/day. In patients who are elderly, underweight, and with poor appetites, protein intake should not be restricted as this can cause **malnutrition**. Are you beginning to see why this is so controversial, and difficult? Malnutrition with a low serum albumin has been associated with a poor prognosis in dialysis patients. If a patient is of normal body weight, a moderate protein restriction should be followed. Patients should also follow a low sodium diet (<2 grams of sodium per day). If kidney function is poor, with less than 30 percent of kidney function, the patient may also need to decrease the amount of phosphorus in the diet. Phosphorus is found in dairy products. You should discuss this with your kidney doctor. Patients with advanced kidney disease often cannot excrete their potassium adequately in the urine and may need to follow a low potassium diet. Some of the foods that contain high levels of potassium include tomatoes, bananas, potatoes, melons, and oranges. There are no other specific dietary recommendations to prevent worsening of kidney disease. Table 3 shows foods that contain high, moderate, and low potassium. Table 4 shows foods that are high in phosphorus.

Malnutrition

Poor nutritional status due to deficiencies in the diet.

Table 3: Foods that contain high, moderate, and low potassium

High potassium (avoid)	Moderate potassium (limit)	Low potassium (incorporate in diet)
All meats, poultry, and fish are high in potassium.	Apple juice	Apples
	Asparagus	Bell peppers
	Beets	Blueberries
Apricots (fresh more so than canned)	Blackberries	Cabbage
	Broccoli	Cranberries
Avocado	Carrots	Cranberry juice
Banana	Cherries	Cucumber
Cantaloupe	Corn	Fruit cocktail
Honeydew	Eggplant	Grapes
Kiwi	Grapefruit	Green beans
Lima beans	Green pears	Iceberg lettuce
Milk	Loose-leaf lettuce	Mandarin oranges, canned
Oranges and orange juice	Mushrooms, fresh	
	Onions	Mushrooms
Potatoes (can be reduced to moderate by soaking peeled, sliced potatoes overnight before cooking)	Peach	Peaches, canned
	Pears	Pineapple, fresh
	Pineapple	Plums
	Raisins	
Prunes	Raspberries	
Spinach	Strawberries	
Tomatoes	Summer squash, including zucchini	
Vegetable juice	Tangerines	
Winter squash	Watermelon	

Table 4: Phosphorous-containing foods

Milk	Hot chocolate/cocoa
Cheese	Bran, oat, or whole wheat cereals
Soda particularly colas	Whole grain bread
Ice cream	Peanut butter
Chocolate	Brown rice
Cookies	Processsed meats, fish, or poultry

61. Are there any specific medications that can prevent my kidney function from getting worse?

If we knew of a medication that would achieve this, both authors would be retired and sipping mint juleps in a Southern locale, living off the rewards of our inventive labors. The short answer is that most of the time our biggest goal is to slow down the almost inevitable loss of kidney function. Preventing it from getting worse is still more in the Disney domain than the real world.

So now that we have revealed the bad news that there are no specific medications that can protect your kidney function forever, or prevent kidney function from getting worse, there is some god news. There are several medications currently available which have been shown to slow the progression of chronic kidney disease. These include using an ACE-inhibitor or ARB (angiotensin receptor blocker), particularly when there is protein in the urine. In some circumstances, when a patient still has a significant amount of protein present in the urine after one of these drugs has been added, it may be necessary to use both an ACE-inhibitor and an ARB together. It is also important to control blood pressure to levels of 130/80 mm Hg in all patients with underlying kidney disease. Sadly, this often means that patients will require 3–4 medications (sometimes even more that) to get to the target blood pressure. Other measures to prevent worsening of kidney function include treatment of high cholesterol usually with a statin drug, aiming to get **LDL** levels (bad cholesterol) to values less than 100 mg/dL. The value of statin treatment has not been shown in a **double blind study** with kidney function loss being the object of the study. Virtually all of the completed statin research studies have specifically lowered cholesterol for the sake of preventing heart disease and stroke. Sifting through those studies, there does seem to be a signal that kidney function is a little better in those that get the real deal (the statin) compared with the sugar pill (placebo.)

LDL

A lipoprotein that transports cholesterol in the blood; composed of a moderate amount of protein and a large amount of cholesterol; high levels are thought to be associated with increased risk of coronary heart disease and atherosclerosis. LDL cholesterol is also known as the "bad" cholesterol and a high level in the blood is thought to be related to various pathogenic conditions.

Double blind study

A clinical study in which neither the participants nor the researchers know which participants are assigned to a certain treatment group.

If a patient is diabetic, his or her blood sugar also needs to be tightly controlled, aiming to reach a target **hemoglobin A1C** of < 7.0. A low protein diet is also sometimes recommended. Patients should also avoid medications that can be harmful to the kidney function, including NSAIDs and contrast dye. Other medication dosages may need to be adjusted for your level of kidney function, so it is best to consult your physician before taking any new medications.

Hemoglobin A1C

Measured in the blood of diabetics to assess long-term sugar control by measuring glycosylated hemoglobin.

62. If I drink a lot of water will this flush my kidneys and prevent the kidney function from getting worse?

There is a perception that drinking 8 glasses of water per day can help maintain normal kidney function. Unfortunately, that is (from what we currently know) exactly what it is: a perception. It is *not* true and usually we would only recommend drinking the amount of fluid required to quench your thirst. High fluid intake does not protect the kidneys. Don't sell the Poland Spring® stock just yet.

In certain circumstances, such as kidney stones, high fluid intake is encouraged to help prevent the formation of new kidney stones.

In certain circumstances, such as kidney stones, high fluid intake is encouraged to help prevent the formation of new kidney stones. Patients often gauge their kidney function from the amount of urine they pass. Volume of urine in general is not related to the amount of kidney function. Even with advanced kidney disease a person may still pass a lot of urine, though the urine may be very dilute and not be filtering the poisons from the kidney. It's an advantage if a patient has worsening kidney function and still passes a lot of urine since it usually helps prevent fluid from accumulating in the body. If you are a patient with kidney disease, you should also be aware that drinking large amounts of a sport fluid such as Gatorade®, which has high electrolyte content, causes an elevation of potassium levels in the blood, which is not usually a good thing.

63. I was told I had a blockage of my kidney and required a stent. What does this mean?

Semantics first: we are sticklers for that. The kidneys can be blocked up in several ways. Their blood flow may be blocked, or their urine flow may be blocked. We will assume you are talking blood flow since **stents** are more commonly used with regard to blood flow.

One cause of kidney disease is due to blockage of blood flow of the main kidney arteries to one or both kidneys. Each kidney usually has one main artery bringing blood to it, but exceptions to that rule are sometimes seen. Blockage of this main artery is usually found in elderly patients with other **vascular** disease (**peripheral vascular disease**—poor blood flow or circulation to usually the lower legs, myocardial infarction or previous heart attack, stroke, disease of the carotid arteries). Such patients often have diabetes, a history of current or prior cigarette smoking, and high cholesterol. There is no current consensus as to what the best treatment is for these blockages. It has not been shown in studies that **angioplasty** or opening up the artery with a balloon and placement of a stent, is any better than medical treatment. There is currently a large national government-sponsored trial looking at this very question. Generally, it is probably better to avoid any unnecessary procedures. There are circumstances when angioplasty or opening up these vessels is indicated. If one has significant (>70 percent narrowing) involvement of both renal arteries, if blood pressure is uncontrolled despite multiple medications, or one has intolerance to blood pressure medications, then angioplasty might be appropriate. In general angioplasty effects can be divided into two categories 1) effect on blood pressure and 2) effect on kidney function. Regarding blood pressure, you can usually reduce the patient's blood pressure medication requirement by two drugs. If you are on five medications, the procedure will usually allow the patient to decrease to three blood pressure medications. Regarding kidney function, about 1/3 of patients get worsening of kidney function, about 1/3 stay

Stent
The main purpose of a stent is to counteract significant decreases in vessel or duct diameter by acutely propping open the conduit by a mechanical scaffold or stent.

Vascular
This term refers to blood vessels. It usually, but not always, refers to the artery type of blood vessels in particular.

Peripheral vascular disease
A collator for all diseases caused by the obstruction of large peripheral arteries, which can result from atherosclerosis, inflammatory processes leading to stenosis, an embolism or thrombus formation. It causes either acute or chronic ischemia.

Angioplasty
Vascular intervention in which dye is injected into an artery.

the same, and about 1/3 have some improvement of kidney function. The important things to remember are to aim to keep blood pressure at 130/80 mm Hg or less, treat cholesterol aggressively with a statin, and aim for an LDL level of less than 100. Before a patient has an angioplasty procedure, the authors believe that you are best served by getting an opinion from a nephrologist who is experienced in this area. If you go ahead, it is valuable to know that your procedure is being done at a center with experience. The procedure itself is not without risk. These risks include worsening of kidney function, bleeding complications, and atheroemboli or showering of cholesterol emboli.

64. How does kidney disease affect my blood count? I was told I should be started on erythropoietin shots. What does that involve?

Once again, we in the kidney disease field are giving some competition to our fellow sub-specialists. In this case it has to do with our colleagues in endocrinology. As you know, **endocrinology** refers to things like hormones and glands. Most people are unaware of the fact that the kidney is an endocrine organ. This means it's not unlike your pancreas or your adrenal glands and it makes hormones, too. In this particular case, the hormone is called erythropoietin.

Erythropoietin (which we call "epo" for short) stimulates the bone marrow to make new red blood cells. When a patient has chronic kidney disease with kidney function at less than 60 percent, the kidney does not produce enough epo to make red blood cells and patient can develop anemia of chronic kidney disease. The hormone is now available by prescription and given as an injection to patients who are anemic with hemoglobin levels of less than 10 g/dL. This hormone does not seem to work in a pill or capsule form because the gut system likely degrades the hormone such that it doesn't work when given by the oral route. Not everyone with mild to moderate

Most people are unaware of the fact that the kidney is an endocrine organ. This means it's not unlike your pancreas or your adrenal glands and it makes hormones, too.

Endocrinology

A branch of medicine that specifically deals with disorders of the endocrine system and its specific secretion of hormones.

kidney failure needs epo, but most people with severe kidney failure, particularly if they are on dialysis, do need it.

David's comments:

My body was not producing enough red blood cells. So to treat my anemia, Dr. Cohen prescribed a monthly shot of Aranesp. My hemoglobin rate was around 9 g/dl when I began receiving the medication. Within weeks, the hemoglobin rose to 12 g/dl. This is the magic number my doctor was shooting for. But there is research under way to show a correlation between hemoglobin rates of 14-15 g/dl and heart disease. Keep a close eye on all the important hemoglobin rates. Oh . . . and the part about having a difficult time in convincing the medical insurers as to the need for erythropoietins? Phew!!!!! The cost can reach more than $1,000 a shot, so batten down the hatches and prepare for battle.

65. I was told there are different kinds of erythropoietin agents. What is the difference between the medications, and does it matter which one my doctor prescribes?

Whether or not we like it, variety is a fact of American life. A walk down any supermarket will confirm even to the most skeptical the truth of this statement. Even in medicine, competition exists for medications that fill a particular medical niche. Erythropoietin is no exception in this regard. Moreover, a desire to produce an effective erythropoietin is a powerful stimulus in the pharmaceutical industry because of the relatively high cost of this kind of medication.

Erythropoietin is available in three forms in the United States. As a category these drugs are called erythropoietin stimulating agents (ESAs). There is recombinant human erythropoietin (Epogen® and Procrit®) and darbepoetin (Aranesp®). Epogen and Procrit are usually given every 1–4 weeks in patients with chronic kidney disease depending on the hemoglobin level. These drugs are given 3 times per week if a patient is on dialysis. Aranesp is usually administered once every 4 weeks. These drugs are very expensive and will usually require approval from your medical insurance company. These drugs have also dramatically reduced the number of blood transfusions that patients with chronic kidney disease require. The injections are given with a small needle, similar to the needles used for insulin administration. Patients can be taught to inject at home or they can come to the nephrologist's or hematologist's office to receive the shot. Procrit and Epogen are shorter acting and need to be administered more frequently than Aranesp, which is active in the blood for a longer period of time.

If you have been on one or the other of these agents and have had a look at the cost, don't faint. Don't worry that someone moved the decimal point two places to the right. They didn't. These agents are pricey and can cost more than a $1,000/month (and you thought your plumber was costly!).

66. I have been told that my "epo" shot should be held as my hemoglobin or blood count was too high. What does this mean? I have been feeling more energetic since starting these shots and feel reluctant to miss a shot. What should I do?

Ever hear the old saying "Too much of a good thing can be a problem?" Here is an example where that is true. Our recent experiences, which have been reported in such high profile journals as the *Wall Street Journal*, have emphasized the fact that when the hemoglobin has been driven to too high a level, the benefit can be outweighed by the risk of heart disease. Given the cost of erythropoietin therapy, there has been intense scrutiny both on its usage as well as its benefits. Although we're not sure why, achieving a normal hemoglobin with erythropoietin therapy is not necessarily a good thing. As a result, we have developed target levels of hemoglobin when we administer epo.

The target hemoglobin level recommended is 10–12 g/dL (a normal hemoglobin is around 13–14 in women and 15 or so in men). It is important not to exceed the target hemoglobin level as doing so has been associated with an increase in cardiac events. Two recent studies looked at hemoglobin levels of 11 and compared them to patients with hemoglobin levels of 13.5. Both studies were done using Procrit® as the epo therapy. There was an unexplained increase in cardiac events in the higher hemoglobin group. Patients on these drugs report improved quality of life and increased energy levels with correction of the anemia. It is probably important to hold off when hemoglobin levels exceed 12 g/dL, as there may be risk of an increase in cardiac events. Until we have further studies, we would strongly recommend following this guideline. Another important point is that none of these studies was conducted using Aranesp and it is not clear that you can generalize these results to patients who are receiving Aranesp. There is currently a large worldwide study being conducted with Aranesp.

67. My doctor's office called to say I need an iron infusion. Is this necessary?

Building new red blood cells requires a few raw materials. Besides erythropoietin, you also need iron. One without the other is like having a nut without a bolt. If there is a deficiency in iron it's like having a car with an empty gas tank. Consequently, when we use erythropoietin therapy, we periodically check to be sure that the gas tank is at least half full.

Sometimes, if iron levels are low, the physician needs to exclude other causes of iron deficiency such as gastrointestinal bleeding before starting these drugs. Almost all patients will require oral iron supplementation and some patients may require intravenous iron infusions to maintain iron levels in the blood. Iron is needed to make red blood cells and once patients start these medications they usually become iron deficient.

If there is a deficiency in iron it's like having a car with an empty gas tank.

Taking iron pills is often constipating. As a result, many physicians and patients prefer to receive the iron by a transfusion. Typically, the transfusion is given in 1 to 3 separate infusions. The good news for those of you who have a needle phobia (like Dr. Townsend) is that the infusion of iron saves a few months of oral iron intake. This is because the intestines are relatively belligerent when it comes to absorbing the iron. Typically less than 10 to 20 percent of iron given as a pill is absorbed.

68. I was told I have parathyroid disease due to my kidney disease. What are my parathyroid glands and where are they located?

Well, we're back to that endocrine thing again. Let's start with a brief review of where the **parathyroid glands** are, what they do, and how the kidneys can potentially interfere with these **endocrine glands**.

The parathyroid glands are small glands located in the neck above the thyroid gland. People usually have four parathyroid glands. They are too small for anyone to feel them, even when enlarged. These glands are important in the control of your calcium and in phosphorus metabolism in your body. The parathyroid gland secretes a hormone called **parathyroid hormone (PTH)**, which can be measured in the blood. The parathyroid hormone reacts in response to calcium, phosphorus, and vitamin D levels in your blood. Vitamin D mainly comes from sunlight, is absorbed through your skin, and is converted in the liver to 25 hydroxyvitamin D. This in turn is converted into the active form that your body can use in the kidney. Here 25 hydroxyvitamin D is converted to 1-alpha hydroxyvitamin D. This active form of vitamin D has a direct role in the secretion or blocking of secretion of PTH. In chronic kidney disease, when kidney function decreases to less than 60 percent of kidney function, patients will often become vitamin D deficient due to inability to convert vitamin D into the active form. In turn, this stimulates the parathyroid gland to become overactive and increase the

Parathyroid glands

Small endocrine glands in the neck, usually located behind the thyroid gland, which produce parathyroid hormone. In rare cases the parathyroid glands are located within the thyroid glands. Most often there are four parathyroid glands, but some people have six or even eight.

Endocrine glands

Glands that secrete specific hormones, which have a specific effect on specific organs; for example, insulin is secreted by the pancreas and is responsible for metabolism of glucose.

Parathyroid hormone (PTH)

A hormone that is secreted from the parathyroid gland and controls the body's metabolism of calcium and phosphorus and is involved in bone metabolism.

secretion of PTH. High levels of PTH are dangerous and can cause severe bone disease with decrease in the calcium content in the bone. Elevated PTH can also cause increase in calcium and phosphorus binding in the blood and this calcium/phosphate product can be deposited in the vessels causing an increase in calcification, or hardening, of the vessels. This may be one factor that contributes to the increase in cardiac risk in patients with chronic kidney disease.

69. Even though my doctor said I have parathyroid disease, I feel well and have no symptoms. Should I take the treatment she prescribed? What is active vitamin D?

When the kidney function becomes sluggish, it forces the parathyroid glands into overtime in their quest to manage the calcium and phosphorus levels in the body. This overactivity in the parathyroid glands, when it's a consequence of kidney disease, is called "secondary hyperparathyroidism." Try saying that six times fast!

One of the partner functions of the kidney, from an endocrine standpoint, is the production of "active" vitamin D. We have a big long name for this: one-alpha-twenty-five-dihydroxy-vitamin D. Maybe that's why we call it "active" vitamin D? In any case, the kidney is responsible for the final steps in producing vitamin D in its active form. As kidneys fail, they relinquish this part of their job description fairly early in the course of kidney disease. As a result, we often give vitamin D supplements to patients with chronic kidney disease as this question covers.

Most patients with **secondary hyperparathyroidism** (or **SHPT** for short) due to vitamin D deficiency from chronic kidney disease do not have any symptoms. It is often a challenge to get patients to take these medications when they have no symptoms and don't feel any different when taking the medications. The problem with SPHT is that it can cause

Secondary hyperparathyroidism (SHPT)

Stimulation of the parathyroid glands due to vitamin D deficiency in chronic kidney disease.

Calcification

Excess deposition of calcium usually in blood vessels.

severe bone disease with increased risk of fracture and bone pain as well as increased risk of **calcification** of the blood vessels. This increases your risk of cardiac events such as heart attack. First line therapy is with active vitamin D since it does not need conversion in the kidney to become active. It is important to realize that the over-the-counter vitamin D contains the form of vitamin D that needs conversion in the kidney. If you have chronic kidney disease, you will not be able to use this source of vitamin D. You will need a prescription from your kidney doctor and he or she will monitor PTH levels every 3–4 months. As kidney disease worsens, calcium levels will decrease due to decreased absorption of calcium from your GI tract since you need active vitamin D to properly absorb it. You also get high levels of phosphate, mainly due to decreased excretion of phosphate by the kidney into the urine. You doctor may also recommend a low phosphate diet and phosphate binders. Phosphate is mainly found in dairy products such as milk products and chocolate. Phosphate binders are used to literally bind phosphate in your GI tract so that you have decreased absorption of phosphate into the blood. There are various phosphate binders available and you should discuss the different phosphate binders with your kidney doctor.

70. I have chronic kidney disease. Can my kidneys get better?

This question is fairly late in the book for a good reason. The brief answer is contained in this paragraph. If we started out our book with such a pessimistic approach to answering questions, you might have read the first questions in the bookstore, or on line, and decided "Wow, there's no hope" and went on to some other purchase. After reading the next paragraph, be sure to read the following one, too.

Unfortunately the kidney is unlike other organs that can regenerate and repair tissues. Once there is chronic kidney disease, it is irreversible and kidney function does not improve.

The goal of your kidney doctor is to stabilize your kidney disease and to try preventing worsening of your kidney disease.

Before you dig out the Prozac, let's stop and talk for a moment. In the authors' opinion, the most important thing about chronic kidney disease is recognizing that it's present, since much can be done to slow the progression to further kidney function loss. Some folks get immobilized by bad news, but others find encouragement in the fact that doctors, nurses, dietitians, health care workers, and patients are all linked through the National Kidney Foundation and the American Association of Kidney Patients. This helps you to keep on top of the problem and develop ways to cope with the presence of CKD and to use every available resource to slow its progression. If anything, having CKD gives one an impressive understanding of just how important the kidneys are in health and wellness.

71. Are there any medications I should avoid if I have kidney disease?

The simple answer is "Yes, most of them!" You should avoid them because they are eliminated by the kidney. If the kidney function is impaired, there is a chance they will accumulate to a higher degree in the bloodstream. Fortunately, the FDA is aware of such things and usually requests a drug manufacturer to give dosing guidance to prescribing doctors and other providers when the patient's kidney function is impaired. The liver is the other organ responsible for metabolizing medication. If you have kidney *and* liver trouble it's even harder to figure out what to do. In some cases, a modest buildup of a drug (like one that lowers blood pressure, for example) would not be likely to do much more than lower your blood pressure a little more. Some drugs have a narrow therapeutic window and they are the ones where dosage adjustment for kidney function is most important. Moreover, if your kidney function is impaired, we often recommend that people avoid certain drugs that are known to cause (in some, but not all people) more kidney function loss.

If you are prescribed any medication, you should always tell your doctor that you have kidney disease. You should also check with your kidney doctor, as many medications need to have the dose adjusted in patients with reduced kidney function. This also includes over-the-counter medications and herbal medications or supplements. Specifically NSAIDs and IV dye or contrast should be avoided. Many other medications including antibiotics and **gout** medications need to have the dosages reduced.

If you are prescribed any medication, you should always tell your doctor that you have kidney disease.

Gout

A disturbance of uric-acid metabolism occurring chiefly in males, characterized by painful inflammation of the joints, especially of the feet and hands, and arthritic attacks resulting from elevated levels of uric acid in the blood and the deposition of urate crystals around the joints. The condition can become chronic and result in deformity.

72. I am overweight and have high blood pressure, diabetes, and chronic kidney disease. Someone suggested I try a high protein diet to lose weight like the Atkins diet. Is this a good idea?

While the authors applaud attempts by patients to try to control weight, in this particular case the Atkins (or other high protein intake) diet is not a good idea. A high protein diet may cause your kidney disease to worsen more rapidly. High protein diets can also precipitate episodes of gout. Most patients with kidney disease should follow a moderately reduced protein diet to help preserve kidney function. It is best to consult with a dietitian regarding specific dietary recommendations including low sodium, low carbohydrate, and moderate protein diet.

So what can you do? Joining a religious order with mandatory fasting periods may appeal to some. That always seems to be problematic for people with diabetes because of the whole insulin thing, as those of you who have suffered through low blood sugar periods will readily testify. There are ways to try to trim back the diet and (hold on, this is going to hurt) exercise more. There's that dreaded "E" word! Think of it from a Newtonian physics standpoint. Why are people overweight? They are overweight because they consume more energy than they use up each day. That was an easy question, wasn't it? Given that premise, how does one go about restoring the balance of calorie expenditure? Keep in mind that each pound of body fat is about 3,500 stored calories. If you want to get rid of a pound of fat, short of liposuction you have to either deny yourself 3,500 calories, or exercise that amount of calories. Isn't physics wonderful? How much exercise would it take if we were to walk off 3,500 calories? Each mile you walk burns about 100. Don't reach for the calculator because this one is easy. (Answer = 35 miles.) Let's see. It takes about an hour for one of the authors (the older one) to walk 4 miles. If he were to walk for nine hours straight (allowing a 15-minute rest), he would lose a pound. No wonder **bariatric** surgery is gaining popularity.

Bariatric
Pertaining to weight.

As to the diet part, the authors believe strongly in the use of a registered dietitian to help. Many agencies like Weight Watchers® have dietitians and, in the long haul, for the sake of your knees, gallbladder, and other valuable body parts that seem to take a hit from being overweight, we think it's very useful to team up with them in the interest of achieving a meaner, leaner, you.

David's comments:

Diet and exercise usually cause low blood sugar episodes in diabetics. Keep an eye on blood sugars even more closely and it's wise to keep a log of your blood sugar numbers. If you continue to experience low blood sugars, make an appointment with your physician and present your log book. The doctor may need to lower your diabetes medications.

73. What is the ideal diet I should follow now that I have been diagnosed with kidney disease?

Glad you asked! Moving right along with the flow from the last question, let's think a little bit more about this one.

The diet should ideally be tailored according to the underlying diseases a patient has. For example, diabetics will have to limit

The diet should ideally be tailored according to the underlying diseases a patient has.

their refined sugar or carbohydrate intake. All patients with CKD should limit their sodium intake to less than 2 grams per day as this will help with blood pressure control and help manage fluid accumulation. There is no specific requirement for fluid intake and you may need to limit fluid intake if you have a tendency to retain fluid. Low to moderate protein in the diet is recommended. You may also need to limit your potassium intake if you have a high potassium level in your blood. Potassium is commonly found in oranges, potatoes, bananas, tomatoes, and melons. A list of potassium contain- ing foods is listed in Table 3 on page 98. You may also need to limit the amount of phosphorus-containing foods in your diet, if your phosphorus level in the blood is high. Phosphorus is found in many foods including dairy products, candy, and sodas. Foods high in phosphorus are shown in the Table 4 on page 98. You should discuss these issues with your kidney doctor and ask for a list of foods to avoid.

74. My doctor said my blood has too much acid and that this is related to my kidney disease. Is there anything I can do to improve this? Is this dangerous?

Those of you who survived the late 1960s may be experienc- ing a flashback right about now. However, it is not *that* kind of acid. To appreciate the answer to this, we need to review some high school chemistry. If you were an English type and hated science, not to worry. We'll use the Cliff Notes® ver- sion herein.

Doctors measure the acid level in the blood by determin- ing the concentration in your blood of a mineral called **bicarbonate**. If that brings to mind the picture of a red circle showing a human arm wielding a big old hammer, bingo— it's the very same stuff. Acid stomach, acid blood, they're related.

Bicarbonate

Alkali content in the blood which is measured with a blood test.

Ideally, the level of bicarbonate in the blood should be about 24 units (where units is meq/L...which is why we said "units"). You get acid from your diet. Once again, recalling those misty days in biology (sorry to be switching around) we were all taught that proteins, like Tinker Toys®, are made up of strings of amino acids. When we eat protein we consume a little bit of acid. When we eat a 12-ounce steak, we consume a fair bit of acid. Only the kidney has the ability to get rid of these kinds of acid. When CKD is present, sometimes the kidney cannot excrete acid effectively and the blood becomes progressively more acidic. This is reflected by the bicarbonate level, which then becomes decreased in your blood. People are usually asymptomatic for a long time, but the increased acid level in your blood does have long-term side effects. Strangely enough, the high acid affects, of all things, the skeleton. This happens because the build-up of acid leaches the calcium from your bone which is used as a buffer for the acid in your blood. Remember putting a chicken bone in vinegar in grade school? Vinegar is mainly acetic acid and the chicken bone loses its calcium into the vinegar and becomes rubbery. This happens, mercifully, to a much lower degree and over a longer period of time, to people.

So how do we spell "relief" here? Your doctor may prescribe something to increase the bicarbonate level in your blood. He or she may prescribe baking soda, which is bicarbonate of soda, and you can take 1–2 tablespoons dissolved in water twice a day. You can also take a liquid sodium bicarbonate called Bicitra; however, the increased sodium may cause you to retain fluid. The biggest problem with Bicitra is that it has a somewhat unpleasant taste. The biggest problem with the bicarbonate given in tablet form or taken dissolved in your favorite fluid or juice is the feeling like your stomach is enlarging. It actually is, since the bicarbonate mixes it up with the stomach acid generating carbon dioxide gas in the process. Both Bicitra and bicarbonate work, though, and your skeleton will thank you.

75. My kidney function is getting worse. My doctor says I need to prepare for dialysis. What does this involve?

Explaining dialysis is one of the longest and most difficult conversations the authors have had with patients. Dialysis is a very scary thing to many people, although every week in the United States about 400,000 people undergo regular dialysis treatments. The lion's share of them have an uneventful time. The best results in a patient undergoing dialysis occur when careful planning about how to get ready for dialysis is undertaken.

Preparation for dialysis should preferably occur at least 6 months prior to a patient starting dialysis. There is a big emotional component when a patient and his or her family need to adjust to the idea of being on dialysis. If a patient is aware and starts preparing for dialysis in advance, there is a far smoother transition to dialysis. Usually when a patient's kidney function is at 20 percent of normal or less, the kidney doctor will start discussing plans for dialysis. There are a number of factors to consider including choosing a type of dialysis, having access placed for dialysis, and listing for transplant. The modalities of each dialysis type will be discussed in the next question. If a patient opts to have **hemodialysis** an appointment with an experienced vascular surgeon should be scheduled. The surgeon will decide if an **arteriovenous fistula (AVF)** can be placed. This is when a native artery and vein are joined together to make a fistula, usually in your forearm, to receive dialysis (see Figure 6). This is a type of vascular access and is the best type of access for a hemodialysis patient to get. The vascular surgeon will usually order **vein mapping** prior to surgery to assess your veins and to plan surgery. Ideally, the AVF should be placed months ahead of a patient needing to start dialysis since it can't be used for 4–6 months while it heals and matures. After an AVF is placed and your wound is healed, you should pump your hand against a stress ball 3–4 times per day for 10 minutes to get the AVF to mature or grow bigger. The AVF is the best choice because it may last many years and rarely becomes

Hemodialysis

Dialysis of the blood to remove toxic substances or metabolic wastes from the bloodstream; used in the case of kidney failure.

Arteriovenous fistula (AVF)

Dialysis vascular access that is surgically created for use to receive dialysis. A native artery and vein are surgically joined together to form the arteriovenous fistula.

Vein mapping

A procedure done with ultrasound which defines the vessels in a patient's arms.

Treatment of Kidney Disease

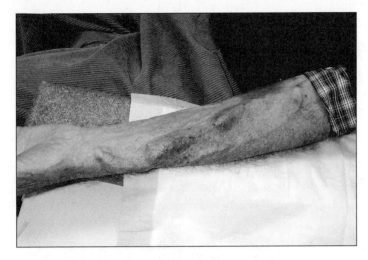

Figure 6. Arteriovenous fistula on a patient's forearm.

infected. This will enable the patient to get the best dialysis and the patient will have a low risk of infection. Occasionally, the surgeon will not be able to find suitable veins and a graft will need to be placed. This is when your own artery and vein are joined together with a synthetic piece of material to form an **arteriovenous graft (AVG)**. The advantages of the AVG are that it can be used for dialysis after about 4 weeks. The disadvantages are that the AVG usually only remains patent, or open, for dialysis for approximately 2 years. It has a higher risk of infection since there is a foreign piece of material in your body. Some patients, like diabetics, with small veins will not be able to have an AVF placed and in these patients an AVG is a good option. If dialysis is not planned ahead of time, the patient may need a tunneled dialysis catheter placed under the skin below the collar bone, which can be used immediately. A **tunneled dialysis catheter** is not a good option since there is a high risk of infection and the quality of dialysis available is poorer. Tunneled dialysis catheters should be reserved for emergencies. The differences between the different vascular accesses options are shown later in Table 6. If you opt to have **peritoneal dialysis (PD)** the patient will need a PD catheter placed at least 2 weeks before dialysis is required. The patient

Arteriovenous graft (AVG)

Dialysis vascular access when a synthetic piece of foreign material is used to join an artery to a vein to create a vascular access.

Tunneled dialysis catheter

A permanent catheter that is inserted usually into the internal jugular vein in order to receive dialysis.

Peritoneal dialysis

Peritoneal dialysis works on the principle that the peritoneal membrane that surrounds the intestine can act as a natural semipermeable membrane and that if a specially formulated dialysis fluid is instilled around the membrane then dialysis can occur, by diffusion.

usually needs to wait 2 weeks for the skin to heal around the catheter site so fluid will not leak. Another important option to consider, once kidney function decreases to less than 20 percent of kidney function, is to get a transplant evaluation. There are a few different options and the waiting list for a deceased donor or **cadaver transplant** is about 5 years, depending on blood type. Other options include getting a kidney from a relative or even another donor who is not related to you but is willing to donate a kidney and is a blood match. Some patients now get a kidney transplant before they need to start dialysis and this is associated with better outcomes.

Cadaver transplant

Organ is donated from a deceased donor or cadaver donor.

76. What is the difference between peritoneal dialysis and hemodialysis. Should I choose one modality over the other?

There are several key differences between these approaches to clearing the blood by an artificial means. It is helpful to briefly review what's involved in each. A separate 100 Questions book is devoted to the topic of dialysis since it is such a huge area and there are so many people who are on dialysis. The important thing to keep in mind is that there is no right or wrong and that your decision about which type to use is not irrevocable, though it does require work to switch over from one kind to another. Let's explain what is involved in these two approaches.

PD is a type of dialysis that is done through a catheter placed in your belly or abdomen. The peritoneal membrane or lining acts as a barrier. Fluid and wastes diffuse through this barrier and are then transported by the tube out of your body. There are many advantages to PD including that it is done at home and it allows the patient more freedom with both his or her lifestyle and diet. Because you are dialyzing every day, there is less restriction on your diet and fluid intake. There are now automated machines that patients hook up to at night and dialyze while they are sleeping. They only come to the dialysis unit to see the doctor once a month or if they are having a problem. The disadvantages are a real risk of infection in the peritoneum or abdominal compartment. Patients need to be very vigilant about their personal hygiene. This is also a less efficient form of dialysis that does not work well for all patients. PD usually works better in patients whose kidney is still functioning to a small degree. The fluid that is infused into the abdomen also has high amounts of dextrose, or sugar, and can make blood sugars more difficult to control if a patient is diabetic. If you are very overweight, or have had a number of previous abdominal surgeries, you may not be a good candidate for PD. This is often a good option for younger patients who are leading an active life, are working, and do not want to be restricted to coming to the dialysis unit 3 times per week.

Hemodialysis (HD) is the more common type of dialysis and is performed by circulating your blood through a filter or **dialyzer**. The advantage of this type of dialysis is that the patient does not have to be actively involved in the dialysis, which may be a good option for older patients who are more frail and less able to be actively involved in their care. Hemodialysis is usually performed in a dialysis center 3 times per week. Some patients may even need to have dialysis 4 times per week. There are some centers that perform dialysis nightly. This is called nocturnal dialysis but is still rarely done in the United States. Disadvantages of this type of dialysis are that a patient is unable to travel unless it is planned in advance, it is time consuming, and most patients require 4 hours of dialysis per treatment. In larger, more muscular patients it can take longer. Patients are also more restricted in their fluid and dietary intake. Most patients will have complete or nearly complete loss in urine output after they start dialysis. Any fluid that is consumed cannot be excreted between treatments and most patients have to severely limit their fluid intake. Patients also need to limit potassium and phosphate intake. HD can now be done at home and this is starting to increase in the United States. Patients or family members are trained to perform the dialysis at home and there are different dialysis prescriptions. Some patients dialyze daily, some at night, and some for a few hours most days of the week. More

Dialyzer

The filter that is used to filter waste products and fluid during the hemodialysis process.

frequent dialysis is associated with improved blood pressure control and less dietary restriction. Home HD is likely to gain popularity in the coming years in younger patients who are independent and want to actively participate in their care.

At our dialysis program at the University of Pennsylvania (and we're pretty similar to other programs throughout the United States) about 90 percent of our dialysis patients receive hemodialysis and about 10 percent are on PD. Differences in hemodialysis and peritoneal dialysis are shown in Table 5.

Table 5: Differences between hemodialysis and peritoneal dialysis

Hemodialysis	Peritoneal Dialysis
Dialysis is performed by circulating your blood through a filter attached to a dialysis machine	Dialysis is performed through your peritoneal membrane in your abdomen
Performed 3 times per week for approximately 4 hours	Performed nightly with automated machine
Dialysis performed by nurse or technician	Patient responsible for own dialysis
Needs to limit fluids and potassium- and phosphorus-containing foods	Less fluid restriction and more liberal diet as dialyzing daily
Difficult to travel as needs to be arranged in advance	Can travel with peritoneal dialysis machine, can get delivery of dialysate supplies throughout the United States
Low risk of infection if patient has arteriovenous fistula or graft	High risk of infection of the peritoneum, need very high level of sterility
No increase in blood sugar	High sugar content of dialysate can make sugar control difficult for diabetics
Need vascular access placed 4–6 months in advance	Can have peritoneal catheter placed 2 weeks before requiring dialysis

77. My doctor says it is a good idea to get a vascular access placed in advance of needing dialysis. How soon do I need to do this? Are there different options?

Ideally, an arteriovenous fistula (or AVF for short) should be placed about 6 months in advance of starting dialysis. You can think of an AVF as a kind of "short circuit" in the blood vessel system. Most of the time, blood goes down arteries, through a capillary bed where it gives up nutrients and picks up wastes, then returns to the heart through the veins. When an AVF is created by a surgeon, it bypasses the capillary and connects the artery (arterio) directly to the vein (venous) through an artificial channel called a fistula. Even though these are usually constructed near the wrist, "fistula" has nothing to do with the "'fist" other than being a nearby neighbor.

It is often difficult to predict exactly when a patient will require dialysis and timing is a difficult decision. If a patient is unable to have an AVF placed due to small peripheral veins we sometimes resort to an arteriovenous graft (or AVG for short). An AVG needs to be placed ideally about 4–6 weeks in advance of starting dialysis.

As a last resort, when time is of the premium and we need to get dialysis going in a very short period of time (like a day or less), a tunneled dialysis catheter is placed temporarily. These are usually discouraged and should really only be placed in an emergency; however, they can be used immediately and can be lifesaving.

If you opt to have peritoneal dialysis you usually need a PD catheter placed about 2 weeks before starting dialysis. This gives the two small wounds involved a chance to get a leg up on healing. Once the PD catheter is in place and you are back up and around, you will usually be taught how to do PD by spending parts of every day for 1–2 weeks at a dialysis training center. Different types of venous accesses for hemodialysis are shown in Table 6.

Table 6: Different vascular access for hemodialysis

Arteriovenous fistula (AVF)	Arteriovenous graft (AVG)	Dialysis catheter
Need 4–6 months before it can be used	Need 4–6 weeks before this can be used for dialysis	Can use immediately
Very low risk of infection	Slightly higher risk of infection as have foreign material in your arm	High risk of infection
Can be used for many years for dialysis	Can usually be used for 2 years before needs replacement	May need to be exchanged often if blood flow is poor
Need to have good vessels, can be a problem in diabetics	Is good access for patients with poor vessels	Do not need good peripheral vessels but can result in clotting of vessel in neck and may not be able to be used again
Able to have high blood flow during dialysis and achieve efficient clearance of toxins	Able to have high blood flow during dialysis and achieve efficient clearance of toxins	Cannot achieve high blood flows and less efficient dialysis

78. Is it true you can do hemodialysis at home? What does this involve?

When dialysis was first done in the United States in the late 1960s, many of the few patients who were fortunate enough to be treated by dialysis did the procedure at home. In 1971, there were about 5,000 people in the United States on dialysis and a lot of them were doing all the necessary stuff at home. Once dialysis treatments became more widely available after 1972, many dialysis centers opened up and home hemodialysis became very uncommon. But, like Dylan said, "the times are a changin'" and home hemodialysis (HHD) is (re)gaining popularity in the United States. HHD is an opportunity for a patient to have the advantage of having HD and also enabling the patient to retain independence and have an active role in their management.

Home HD is ideal for younger, more healthy patients or patients who have an excellent family support system. Home HD involves an intensive training course when either the patient or a dedicated family member is taught to dialyze the patient at home, including how to stick the vascular access and how to troubleshoot the dialysis machines. There are varying prescriptions for home HD. They include daily dialysis for a few hours, nocturnal dialysis, or dialyzing for 3–4 hours 4–5 times per week. Overall, most home HD patients are highly motivated and have a larger dialysis dose delivered. This has been associated with improved blood pressure and less fluid retention. There are specific programs in the United States that train patients to do home HD. The dialysis company also provides 24-hour assistance and a help line for technical problems.

79. My doctor said I can't take NSAIDs for my arthritis as this can make my kidney function worse. Is this true, and is there an alternative to treat my arthritis pain?

It is true, alas. Alternatives are limited and we suggest three things to consider.

First, this is generally true for patients with CKD. NSAIDs can cause worsening of kidney function in a number of different ways. Some of the effects are temporary and can be reversed if stopped early enough while others cause progressive worsening of kidney function. So, in the best of circumstances, patients with CKD should completely avoid NSAIDs and use acetaminophen-based products for pain.

Second, one of the authors (again the *older* one) has experienced yet another of life's rewards for growing older. In this instance, it's an entity with the dubious distinction of being called a "frozen shoulder." In the process of dealing with this, the words "physical therapy" have changed from something he recommended to patients without ever having had himself, to something that, though actually quite painful, is yielding some rewards in terms of day to day pain reduction and increased mobility. It may be that you could benefit from some physical therapy and some dedicated exercises to change the manner in which we place life's daily wear and tear needs on our joints.

Third, it is sometimes the case that an alternative to medication or physical therapy can help. In this case, we're talking about acupuncture which does indeed help some people with pain. Alternatively, a chiropractor may be of benefit. As the authors age and experience more and more limits on what conventional medical treatment has to offer, we have become increasingly mindful of the role of our allied health brethren in soothing the many ills patients suffer.

Some things (like large doses of vitamin A) can build up to toxic levels in people with kidney function impairment.

One cautionary word is the use of megadoses of vitamins and other supplements. Check with your docs before you consume these things. They may be fine and they may even help, but some things (like large doses of vitamin A) can build up to toxic levels in people with kidney function impairment.

80. My doctor said I should list for a kidney transplant because my kidney function is getting worse. What does this mean?

Physicians, like many professionals, tend to have a vocabulary all their own. When the older author lived in Pittsburgh, he learned a little Pittsburghese, which has stuck with him to this day. He still says "pop" when he means "soda"; "gum bands" when he means "rubber bands" and occasionally there is that problem with infinitives when he says "this needs changed" instead of "this needs to be changed." In this question is another example of provincial terminology where we say a person needs to "list" for a transplant. This is a medieval term, harking back to days of yore when knights placed their names on a list for a tournament and were said to have "entered the list" or "been listed" and waiting their turn. Those of you listed for transplant, know that once listed you may be waiting years for your turn. So when does one "list up"?

When your kidney function decreases to 20 percent of normal or less you can list for a **deceased donor transplant (DDT)** or cadaver kidney transplant (recall from Question 14 that this means an eGFR around 20 mL/min/1.73m²). The **United Network for Organ Sharing** (UNOS; the watchdog organization that oversees kidney transplants in the United States) only allows patients with CKD to list for a DDT when kidney function has decreased to this level. Type 1 diabetics can be listed for DDT when their level of kidney function decreases below 30 percent. It is important to be evaluated and get listed for a kidney transplant as soon as kidney function deteriorates to this level. There are many patients in the United States waiting for a kidney transplant with much fewer donors than those on the waiting list. Currently, there are approximately 77,000 patients waiting for a kidney donation in the United States and most patients will wait 5 years on average for a DDT. The wait time will depend on your blood type and the region where you live. In Pennsylvania, on average, patients with blood type AB wait 2 years, blood type A wait 3–4 years, blood type B wait 4–6 years, and blood type O wait approximately 5 years. Once you are referred for a kidney transplant, you will need to undergo extensive testing to make sure that you are a good candidate to receive a transplant. This includes testing for underlying heart disease and cancers. If you pass the stringent testing, you will then be listed for a DDT in your region and will require monthly blood work.

Deceased donor transplant

Organ transplant from a deceased or cadaver donor.

United Network for Organ Sharing (UNOS)

A non-profit, scientific, and educational organization that administers the nation's only Organ Procurement and Transplantation Network (OPTN), established by the U.S. Congress in 1984.

David's comments:

After the smoke clears and you are faced with the reality of transplantation, you must get a battery of tests in order to be placed on the waiting list for a kidney transplant. It's wise to investigate as many locations as possible as the transplant list is sectional. For example, if you are in Philadelphia, you may want to look at New York, Washington, even Florida. After all, you have about a half day or more to act on a transplant. If you are on a list, it might be wise to keep a bag packed with spare essentials, in case you have to hop on a plane. And the other (and much preferred) alternative, the live donor, a family member, or friend who volunteers a kidney. I found it especially difficult to ask for a kidney, until my dear friend Jody put it this way. She said "If your friend or family needed a transplant, how would you feel?" I answered I would jump at the opportunity to help. That certainly put things in perspective and made it much easier to ask. I had a bunch of people step up for me and go through the testing. Luckily my dear cousin, Tony, is a match. He is my hero!!!!

81. My friend has offered me a kidney. How can I find out if my friend is a match? Do you have to be related to receive a kidney from a "live" donor?

With more friends like this the 5-year wait we mentioned in the prior question could be reduced a great deal. Such altruism is rare and greatly valued. Your friend deserves major kudos, but there are hurdles involved in the process. Let's consider a bit more about transplant evaluation to see where the hurdles are located.

Once you have had an evaluation and it has been determined that you are a suitable candidate to receive a transplant from either a deceased or living donor, the options of living donation will be discussed with you. **Living related transplant** is when you are related to the donor, such as your parent, child, or sibling. This is the most common form of living donation and there is increased likelihood of matching or being compatible when you are related to the donor. Living unrelated transplant is gaining popularity. This is when you receive a transplant from a spouse, friend, or sometimes a complete stranger. You must be compatible with the donor to receive

Living related transplant

Organ transplant from a living donor who is related; i.e., is a sibling, parent, or child of the kidney recipient.

the transplant, which means you must have the same blood type or be able to receive a transplant for the donor's blood type. If you are determined to be a good transplant recipient, you can have as many people as needed tested for blood type and if they match further testing will be done. So, the answer is yes, a friend can donate.

We would be remiss if we if we stopped here. There are some ethical considerations involved in the whole organ sharing process. We think its worthwhile to at least mention here that when the situation posed in this question arises, there is a worry that large cash sums could be exchanged for a kidney. You might recall the scandal a few years ago when someone offered one of their kidneys on eBay. Such concerns are likely to come up during a transplant donor evaluation. Don't take it personally if they do. It is part of the job of those doing the evaluating to ensure that there is no evidence of coercion in the process. Donating a kidney is an operation, and though uncommon, there are sometimes complications from operations. Thus, it is the job of those involved in the evaluation process to be thorough and ensure that everything is above board before proceeding.

82. My doctor said that because I have CKD I am at increased risk of cardiac events in the future. Is this true, and why is it true?

This is in fact true. It has been noted that CKD is a risk factor for cardiac events and is now regarded as a risk factor as are high blood pressure or smoking. This means that having CKD does put you at an increased risk of having a heart attack, heart failure, or stroke. We don't really understand why it is so. There is a large amount of research being done to try to figure out exactly what it is about having an increased creatinine that increases your risk of cardiac disease. One group doing such research is the CRIC study group (www.cristudy.org) to which both authors belong.

Until we have further answers to this specific question, it is very important to control for the factors that we know are normally associated with increased cardiac risk. This includes good control of blood pressure with goal blood pressure of 130/80 mm Hg or less, good control of cholesterol with goal LDL of less than 100 mg/dL, good blood sugar control if diabetic with goal Hgb A1C of 7.0 percent or less (but not too much less according to the latest information), smoking cessation, increased aerobic activity, and weight loss.

PART SEVEN

Kidney Stones

I have blood in my urine and very severe pain in my left side. Could I have a kidney stone?

How do I collect a 24-hour urine? Why do I have to do 2 collections on 2 consecutive days?

When should I see a kidney stone specialist?

More . . .

83. I have blood in my urine and very severe pain in my left side. Could I have a kidney stone?

Bloody urine and flank (side) pain have a pretty limited list of possibilities, and kidney stone disease is the first batter in that line-up.

This could very likely be a kidney stone but one always has to keep other diagnoses in mind. Classically, a patient with kidney stones presents with sudden onset of severe pain in either the right or left flank. The pain usually starts in the flank and radiates to the groin in the same direction as the passage of the stone. Patients will usually have some blood in the urine. Pain can be extremely severe and is usually relieved with passage of the stone. Kidney stones often recur and often there is a family history of kidney stones. Patients may also have a history of gout, parathyroid disease, or much less common diseases such as **cystinuria**. Usually a patient with blood in the urine and the classic pain will be presumed to have a kidney stone. A plain X-ray of the abdomen will show if you have a calcium-contianing stone. An ultrasound can be done which will pick up kidney stones as well as obstruction to urine flow if the stone is large and causing obstruction. A CT scan without dye can also be done to assess if a stone is present or if obstruction is present. Patients may require intravenous fluids and pain management until the stone is passed. If the stone is very large (>10mm) or is causing obstruction of urine flow, the stone may have to be removed by either **lithotripsy** or by extracting the stone through the bladder.

The pain in this instance is exquisite. It may come in waves (and is said to have a colic nature). Many say that for men experiencing this, it's the closest they will ever come to understanding what women go through in childbirth.

Cystinuria

An abnormal accumulation of cystine in the urine.

Lithotripsy

The procedure of crushing a stone in the urinary bladder or urethra by means of a lithotriptor, a device that passes shock waves through a water-filled tub in which the patient sits. The resulting stone fragments are small enough to be expelled in the urine.

84. I have had 2 episodes of kidney stones. How do I prevent this from happening again?

It helps a lot to know what the stones were composed of. Most kidney stones are made from calcium, but other things like uric acid and cysteine can form stones in the kidney's collection system. Sometimes you can try to treat underlying disorders (like a lot of calcium being taken out of bone and appearing in the urine because of an overactive parathyroid gland or acid build-up).

Some general measures help, too. Prevention of recurrence of stones is often possible by increasing fluid intake and limiting sodium intake. It is important to increase fluid intake as if taking a prescription. We recommend that patients take ten eight ounce servings or glasses of fluid per day. We suggest 2 8-ounce glasses of fluid with breakfast, lunch, and dinner and another 2 glasses in the late afternoon and 2 glasses before bedtime. Limiting sodium in the diet is important as increased sodium intake is accompanied by increased absorption of calcium and increased likelihood of stone recurrence in the case of calcium stones.

85. I was diagnosed with a kidney stone. My doctor said I must strain my urine to try to collect the stone when I pass it so it can be sent for analysis. Is this important?

If you think back one question, you'll see that for treating kidney stone disease, it is helpful to know a bit about the kidney stone composition. Sometimes stones just happen, but often an underlying cause can be found. Knowing the type of kidney stone helps narrow the search for a cause and guides us along the path to treating it.

Determining the type of stone you have passed is particularly important when it can be used to help prevent recurrence of stones. Most stones are from calcium but many patients also have uric acid stones. The treatment and prevention of these stones are different. If you pass a stone, the doctor will send it off for stone analysis. The stone contents will guide your doctor about further prevention and give useful information on how to prevent further episodes of stones.

There are one or two aids you can think about in this process. For women, there is a "potty insert" that can be placed between the toilet seat and the toilet bowel that will catch urine and has a convenient little spout on it to allow you to pour it through a strainer. Most stones are tiny (we know, why not call them "kidney pebbles" instead of kidney stones? Those of you who have had the experience of passing one of these will think they should have been called "kidney boulders."). They are often not too much bigger than a grain of sand or a small aquarium-sized stone. The hassle of straining for these is worth the effort though. There is nothing like knowing what you're dealing with to deal with it effectively.

86. I have high blood pressure and was recently diagnosed with kidney stones. Is there any BP medication that can help with both problems?

It isn't often that medicine offers a "have your cake and eat it too" scenario, but this is one time when it works out that way. There is a treatment that is ideal both for patients with hypertension and calcium-containing kidney stones. It's a class of drugs known as thiazide diuretics.

Thiazide diuretics are recommended as first line therapy in most patients with uncomplicated hypertension. Thiazide diuretics also result in decreased excretion of calcium in the urine and will decrease formation of calcium stones. Because of that, thiazide diuretics are often the ideal treatment for patients with uncomplicated mild hypertension and calcium containing kidney stones. Best of all they're really cheap, about a penny a pill.

87. I have had several kidney stones, and been told to drink lots of fluids. What type of fluids do I need to drink?

We mentioned increasing fluid intake to include ten eight-ounce glasses of fluid per day. This includes 2 glasses of fluid with each meal, 2 glasses in the late afternoon, and 2 glasses at bedtime. The purpose of the high fluid intake is to continually flush the kidneys and bladder and prevent stone formation; the type of fluid may also be also important. The safest answer to this question is the fluid with the least taste, but the least adulterants too—good ol' water.

Grapefruit juice has been associated with increased risk of calcium stone formation and should be avoided. Coffee and tea have traditionally been thought to increase stone risk due to increased oxalate content. **Oxalate** does not get along too well with calcium in the urine and tends to precipitate the calcium forming the nidus, or center, of a kidney stone. This has not been borne out in research studies but it is probably worthwhile limiting (though not necessarily avoiding) these types of fluids. Excess alcohol should also be avoided since it may increase stone risk. Orange juice may be protective because it contains both potassium and citrate, both of which act like "peacemakers" for minerals like calcium oxalate, which tends to precipitate in urine. There are no definite links with cranberry juice and stone formation. The other fluid we tend to discourage is Gatorade®, mostly because the sodium in it tends to increase the urine calcium excretion.

Oxalate

Oxalate is found in many foods and combines with calcium to form kidney stones.

88. I have had 3 calcium stones. Should I limit the calcium in my diet?

Great question. It would seem like "Duh! Yeah!" would be the answer. Get ready for a surprise ending.

Limiting calcium intake in the diet does *not* decrease your chance of having kidney stones and it is not recommended.

A moderate calcium intake is recommended as research has shown that limiting calcium in the diet may result in an increased chance of developing osteoporosis or weak bones. It does not decrease your chance of developing further calcium stones. Most stones are composed of calcium bonded to oxalate and foods high in oxalate should be avoided (see Table 7). You have to absorb both the calcium and the oxalate for them to make their way through the body in to the urine. One way we think that the findings from research show that calcium intake does not correlate to calcium stone disease is that the calcium in the diet probably binds to the oxalate in the diet. That keeps it from being absorbed in the first place so it gets lost in the stool when you have a bowel movement.

Table 7: Foods to avoid that are high in oxalate

Apples	Asparagus	Beer
Beets	Berries	Black Pepper
Broccoli	Chocolate	Cocoa
Coffee	Cola drinks	Collards
Figs	Grapes	Ice Cream
Milk	Oranges	Parsley
Peanut butter	Pineapples	Swiss Chard
Rhubarb	Tea	Turnips
Vitamin C		

Calcium stone formation is actually more closely linked to sodium intake due to the way calcium is absorbed in your kidney. Limiting sodium intake in the diet is the most important dietary adjustment you can make (thus the Gatorade® or other sodium-fortified beverage response in the prior question).

89. I have a history of gout and recently had a stone that was found to contain uric acid. Is this related to my gout, and how can I avoid this happening again?

Uric acid is one of those minerals in the body that we live with day to day in a cautious balance, much like the détente between the United States and the USSR in the 1970s and 1980s. When both sides behave, a cautious tolerant existence is possible. Unfortunately, uric acid is minimally soluble (like putting sugar into an ice cold glass of tea and waiting forever for the stuff to dissolve) and it doesn't take much to have uric acid declare its nasty little self in an episode of crystal formation in one of three places.

When the body becomes a bit more acidic, uric acid becomes much less soluble and the individual uric acid molecules stick together and grow larger and larger until they become visible crystals. Two such places are in the joint space and the urine, thus gout (in the joint space) and the urine collecting systems are the two places that uric acid build-up causes the most trouble. The third place is in the skin. Uric acid can deposit in the skin in bumps we call "**tophi**" (see tophus in glossary).

Patients with high amounts of uric acid may develop uric acid stones, gouty **arthritis**, or both disorders. The most important way to prevent uric acid stones from recurring is by limiting purines (which come from animal protein) in the diet. This includes red meat, chicken, fish, and red wine. Another way to prevent uric acid stone formation is to **alkalinize** the urine, in other words to make the urine less acidic since acidic urine increases the solubility of uric acid and results in greater stone formation. Managing uric acid kidney stones is a great example of "Better living through chemistry in the home." We typically prescribe sodium citrate or potassium citrate to make

Tophus

(Latin: "stone", plural tophi) is a deposit of crystallized monosodium urate in people with longstanding hyperuricemia. At this stage, most have already developed symptoms of the associated crystal arthopathy known as gout.

Arthritis

Inflammation of the joints.

Alkalinize

To increase the alkali component or the pH in the blood or urine by adding a bicarbonate based agent.

the urine more alkaline. In turn, this increases the solubility of the uric acid in the urine. We often recommend that patients purchase litmus paper to test the urine **pH** and that they can vary the amount and frequency of the potassium citrate to keep a urine pH above 7.0.

pH

pH is a measure of the acidity or alkalinity of a solution.

If uric acid levels are high in the blood, the patient still has recurrent uric acid stones despite the dietary measures listed above and the patient is following an increased fluid intake and urinary alkalinization, we often start treatment with a drug called allopurinol. Allopurinol blocks uric acid production and lowers uric acid levels in the blood.

90. My doctor checked a 24-hour urine as I have a history of recurrent stones. She said my citric acid level in my urine was too low. How do I increase this and why is this important?

You probably noted the similarity between citric acid and citrus fruits. Citric acid is very important in the body's biochemistry and is used in all sorts of cell processes. A certain amount of citrate is excreted in the urine, and this citrate gets between calcium and things like oxalate like a referee at a boxing match. By keeping the "contenders" (calcium and oxalate, for example) apart, there is less formation of kidney stones.

Citric acid is generally checked by collecting a 24-hour urine specimen and measuring how much is lost in the urine over a day and a night. When your citric acid levels are low in the urine, you have increased likelihood of forming stones. We don't usually dwell on why the citrate levels are low, since it is pretty easy to replenish the citrate with a supplement. Consequently, patients with recurrent stones and low citric acid are usually prescribed potassium citrate such as Urocit-K®, which increases the citrate in the urine and reduces the chance of stone formation.

91. How do I collect a 24-hour urine? Why do I have to do 2 collections on 2 consecutive days?

You would think that collecting urine for 24 hours would be cumbersome but straightforward. Of all the things we ask patients to do, this is one that no matter how much effort we go into, and how many well-written handouts we give them, there is a significant chance that the urine will be collected incorrectly. Let's first review what's involved and then do some troubleshooting.

It is important to collect the 24-hour urine correctly. Usually, patients do not collect all the urine in the 24-hour period and this can result in incorrect interpretation of the results. When collecting a 24-hour urine, you must discard the first urine specimen on the first day. Then you must collect all urine for the next 24 hours *including* the first urine specimen on the 2nd day. The urine should be kept in the refrigerator. We know that's unpleasant. Keep it in a double wrapped brown paper bag and *don't* invite your gossipy relatives over during the time you are collecting it unless you enjoy grossing folks out! You should follow your regular diet and fluid intake when collecting a specimen so this can reflect your usual diet and practices. Recommendations will then be based on this collection. It is important to do two collections of urine as one urine jug contains acid as a preservative and certain of the substances are specifically measured in this type of urine while other substances need to be collected without preservative.

Troubleshooting tip #1. If you get up and pee during the night—it goes into the jug.

Troubleshooting tip #2. When you get up in the morning, the urine you pass at your finish time *goes into the jug.*

Troubleshooting tip #3. If you need to have a bowel movement, urinate first, then have the bowel movement.

Troubleshooting tip #4. (This one is for extra credit!) Place a paper bookmark in front part of your underwear to remind you to collect the urine, especially if you are out and about. It sounds weird, but it works. This last one is courtesy of the authors' good friend and colleague Dr. John Daugirdas.

92. I heard there is a special collection kit that avoids you having to send in all the 24-hour urine and that you can mail the specimen in. What's up with that?

Learning from the folks at FedEx and others that successfully cater to clients, there is now a system in place called Litholink, which allows the patient to collect 24-hour urines at home but only requires the patient to send in a small specimen from that 24-hour urine collection. There is a service that picks up the urine from your home and then transports it for analysis. A detailed report is then sent to your doctor with specific recommendations. For more information go to www.litholink.com.

93. When should I see a kidney stone specialist?

This is another one of those queries that can get us into trouble since there are no hard and fast rules to answer it. One logical answer is when you have had a recurrence, or several recurrent kidney stones and don't seem to be getting on top of the situation. Some of the answer will depend on how knowledgeable about and how interested in the situation your doctor is.

Kidney stones often recur. Once a male has had one episode of a calcium-containing stone he has a 15 percent chance of having a recurrent stone at 1 year, 30–40 percent chance of having a recurrent stone at 5 years and a 50 percent chance of having a recurrent stone at 10 years. Some recommend that if you have more than two episodes of kidney stones, it is worthwhile for the patient to be evaluated by a kidney stone specialist. Often after one episode of kidney stones, just increasing your fluid intake and limiting the sodium in your diet may be enough to prevent further stone recurrence in the case of calcium kidney stones.

PART EIGHT

Acute Renal Failure

During my hospitalization I had ARF and required several dialysis treatments. Then the doctors said my kidneys were starting to recover and I did not need any more dialysis. How do I know if my kidneys have recovered?

If I had an episode of ARF in the past am I more likely to develop kidney problems in the future?

I had an ultrasound exam of my abdomen and was found to have hydronephrosis of both kidneys and my prostate was found to also be enlarged. What does this mean?

More . . .

94. My family member is hospitalized with pneumonia and was very ill. She was required to stay in the Intensive Care Unit on a ventilator. The doctors said she has "acute renal failure" but should recover her kidney function. What does this mean?

There is a lot going on in this question. The path revolves around the issue of acute kidney failure, or as it is often now called "**acute kidney injury**" or AKI for short. The authors remain amazed at how often this does *not* occur when people are very sick in the hospital. Sometimes, as in this case, there is just more load than the kidneys can bear and they walk off the job like a disgruntled employee. This is sometimes heralded by a dramatic reduction in urine volume and almost always an increase in the blood level of creatinine.

Acute renal failure (ARF) is common in hospitalized patients who are sick enough to require ICU care. Often, these patients are extremely ill and require ventilator assistance and medication to support the blood pressure. These patients often develop ARF, which may be reversible if the patient recovers from their acute illness. Kidney function can return back to normal or baseline meaning a return to the kidney function that the patient had before the acute illness. The most common cause of ARF is **acute tubular necrosis (ATN)** and this form of ARF is usually reversible. However, there are other types of ARF that are not so reversible and kidney function continues to get worse. Fortunately this type of ARF is not that common.

The biggest hurdle faced in these cases is that for the kidneys to heal the patient has to survive. You are often looking at a few weeks for this to come about.

95. During my hospitalization I had ARF and required several dialysis treatments. Then the doctors said my kidneys were starting to recover and I did not need any more dialysis. How do I know if my kidneys have recovered?

Being in the hospital exposes you to almost futuristic technology at this time. Despite all the fancy trappings attending a hospital experience, the answer to this question is, by contrast, actually very simple. It amounts to two things, as we'll see next.

ARF can be severe enough to require dialysis during a hospital stay. The patients often do recover renal function. Some patients may only require 1–2 dialysis treatments while others may require multiple treatments for weeks or even months before there is recovery of renal function. Usually in patients with ARF, the nephrologists will assess the patient daily and assess the need for dialysis. Once the kidneys start to recover, the patient will often not require further dialysis. Recovery of renal function is monitored by following the urine output carefully which will usually start to increase with recovery of renal function. The nephrologist will also monitor the serum creatinine levels and once creatinine levels are decreasing on their own, and not because of dialysis usually in conjunction with increasing urine output, the nephrologist will hold dialysis. The doctor will then observe the patient for a few days to make sure recovery of renal function continues and the patient no longer requires dialysis.

Acute Renal Failure

96. I had an episode of acute renal failure while in the hospital for heart valve replacement surgery. When I left the hospital the doctor said my kidney function had "slipped a little" but was "returning to baseline." What does this mean, and will this affect my kidney function in the long term?

As we've hopefully indicated by now, you can't tell how well your kidneys are doing until they are doing so poorly that you have become uremic. While in the hospital, it is not uncommon to have short-lived increases in the blood creatinine level that indicate that some loss of function has occurred (or slipped) but you may not have noticed anything at all. Sometime it is because of fluctuations in blood pressure, medications, CT scans, etc. If the creatinine increase is small (usually less than 1 mg/dL increase; going, for example, from 1.2 mg/dL to 2.0 mg/dL) nephrologists are often not called in for consultation as such increases are usually "short term" and often get better on their own.

"Baseline" kidney function is the level of kidney function that you had prior to having the ARF. You can get acute renal failure on top of previously normal kidney function or on top of chronic kidney disease. Baseline kidney function may not be normal kidney function and usually the nephrologist (if one is called into the case) will try to track down your old medical records to see what your prior kidney function was. We generally expect that kidneys will not improve any further than the baseline. Your long-term kidney function depends on the underlying cause of ARF. ARF is usually reversible and will typically return to baseline when the underlying cause of ARF is due to:

1. An obstruction to urinary flow that is relieved.

2. A case of mild acute tubular necrosis, the most common type of ARF in hospitalized patients.

3. ARF due to certain medications may be reversible in some cases but certain medications such as amphotericin B (used for severe infections with fungi) may result in irreversible loss of kidney function.

4. ARF due to IV contrast is usually reversible as well.

5. Allergic reaction of the kidney to medications is usually reversible if detected early.

6. Atheroemboli causing ARF is not reversible. You should discuss this in detail with your kidney doctor.

Most people in the situation described by this question are nearly back to their baseline creatinine value. For example, if you were 1.6 mg/dL and underwent your valve surgery increasing to 3.0 mg/dL, you might have shown creatinine values of 2.6 mg/dL two days ago, 2.2 mg/dL yesterday and 2.0 mg/dL today. In that case, it would be expected that you would gradually return to your 1.6 mg/dL baseline. You would not need to remain hospitalized for that to occur since there is nonspecific treatment we give that hastens the return of kidney function.

97. If I had an episode of ARF in the past am I more likely to develop kidney problems in the future?

This is a very important question, and there is not a lot of information available on which to base an answer. It is such an important issue, though, that the portion of the US government that sponsors much of the medical research done in the United States (the National Institutes of Health) has issued a request for research study proposals that specifically address this area. What we can say is, and we know we tend to sound repetitive, this depends on the cause of ARF. In most cases, it is due to an acute episode of illness or due to medication or toxin and is usually reversible. If you recover kidney function, it does not affect your long-term kidney function and this does not predispose you to getting kidney problems in the future.

98. I have an enlarged prostate and was seen in the ER where I was found to have renal failure related to the enlarged prostate. What does this mean and how can I treat it?

Another very common consequence of aging in men is the development of this particular problem. Part of why it's so problematic is that it comes on very slowly and thus is often present for a long time before it gets so severe that someone is forced, by illness, to have it evaluated and treated.

An enlarged prostate can cause obstruction to urine flow from the bladder. This can result in ARF or CKD or both. This is usually reversible if caught early enough without any effect on long-term kidney function. Sometimes the use of medications for cough/cold/flu symptoms worsens the obstruction and brings the prostate problem into the limelight when a man cannot urinate despite an increasingly impatient urge to do so. The treatment involves relieving the obstruction usually by inserting a bladder (or Foley) **catheter**. For a long-term solution, the prostate size needs to be reduced. This can be achieved with medications or several different types of surgeries. Prostate cancer always needs to be considered as a cause of an enlarged prostate. How this kind of problem is discovered is answered in the next question.

Catheter

A tube that can be inserted into a body cavity.

99. I had an ultrasound exam of my abdomen and was found to have hydronephrosis of both kidneys and my prostate was found to also be enlarged. What does this mean?

Once again a lengthy medical term reveals its simplicity when broken down into component parts. "**Hydronephrosis**" has two component parts. Let's start with the first one: "hydro" or water. That was pretty simple. What about nephrosis? We have seen that "nephro" refers to the kidney and in medical terms any "-osis" is a condition or state of something. So put-

Hydronephrosis

Distention and dilation of the renal pelvis, usually caused by obstruction of the free flow of urine from the kidney.

ting these pieces together we have a state where there is water in the kidney. We know that urine is mostly water so what makes this different from normal? The "amount" of water is the answer. Although urine collects into the system which drains each kidney into the bladder, the system is made in such a way that you don't even notice its doing such a great job. When you look into the system with an ultrasound beam, it paints a nice picture of the kidney as shown in the left side of Figure 5. On the right, you can see a much larger black area representing the collection of urine (water) that is now stretching, or distending, the collection system and causing a water (hydro-) kidney (-nephro-) condition (-osis). A brief anatomical tour is up next after which we will (finally) actually answer this question.

The kidneys channel the urine into the bladder through the ureters. The bladder in turn connects to the outside world through a single passageway called the urethra. Almost like a turnpike tollbooth, partway along the urethra (but only in men) is wrapped the prostate gland. Normally the size of an unshelled walnut, it doesn't usually cause much trouble before about age 50. After that, for lots of reasons, it can enlarge. The enlarged prostate can cause obstruction to outflow of urine from the bladder and this can result in swelling or enlargement of both kidneys, like a clog in the main drain to a house can cause a back-up in the bathrooms. This is most easily seen on an ultrasound examination. If the obstruction is detected acutely and the urine can drain, it's usually reversible. This is achieved by a bladder catheter which is inserted into the bladder. Long-term solutions are also required to decrease the size of your prostate.

There are two problems that can ensue if this is unnoticed, or left untreated. The first one is a loss of kidney function. Think about flushing the toilet when you know the main hose drain is blocked and you get the idea. Urine seeks ways to leak into the body and waste products begin to build up in the blood. The second problem is one of infection. Anytime there is abnormal fluid collection or backup in the body its open season for passing germs to set up residence. For both reasons, it is important to know about this problem and to do something about it when you are fortunate enough to have had it revealed.

PART NINE

Further
Information

Are there any websites or support groups so that I can learn more about my kidney disease?

Are there any kidney diseases that I should consider having genetic testing done for?

More . . .

100. Are there any websites or support groups so that I can learn more about my kidney disease?

There are many sites available on the Internet for patients to browse for information regarding chronic kidney disease, and patients who have chronic kidney disease that are banded together in a support group. The authors recommend starting with the National Kidney Foundation's website which is located at: www.nkf.org.

From this page choose "Kidney Disease" and you will be taken to another page where the opportunity to cruise various aspects of kidney disease and its care at your leisure.

Another website is sponsored by Revolution Health located at: www.revolutionhealth.com/conditions/kidney-bladder/kidney-disease/?s_kwcid=kidney|853885854

A website specifically devoted to patients with kidney disease is located at: www.aakp.org

This site contains a wealth of information for patients interested in knowing more about chronic kidney disease. The authors receive their publication *Renal Life*. This magazine is published six times a year. The website gives you instructions on how to obtain a complimentary copy to see if the nature of the articles suits your particular needs.

David's comments:

Davita has a wonderful website with plenty of mouthwatering, kidney friendly recipes with photos. http://www.davita.com/recipes/. Bon Appetite!

(Bonus Question—how's that for getting your money's worth?)

101. Are there any kidney diseases that I should consider having genetic testing done for?

We reserve this as the last question just in case a late-breaking story or research finding happened between the time we finished writing this book and its publication. The developments in the genetics field are progressing at a mind-boggling rate. There are a number of genetic tests now available for kidney disease. However, there is no recommendation that says simply because the test is available a person with that kidney disease should have it, and have their children tested as well. The decision to undertake genetic testing has some potential consequences that need to be considered before the blood is drawn, the DNA extracted, and the test performed.

One possible complication is a change in insurability status. If your health-care insurer finds out that your children carry a mutation associated with a particular kidney disease, their ability to someday get insurance on their own could be affected. Moreover, there usually are no cures for genetic disorders so knowing that the gene is present does not really inform treatment. It can inform how often we monitor kidney function and check for known consequences if the genetic issue has multiple effects besides reducing kidney function. There may be room to improve on this in the future, but at the present time gene therapy is still largely a promise more than a reality when it comes to kidney disease.

The authors want to especially emphasize, however, that genetic testing done in a research study is a completely different animal. When we perform genetic testing as part of a research study, we usually treat the samples anonymously. We do this to protect the confidentiality of the findings from discovery by health-care insurers or other agencies. This is legalized by a Certificate of Confidentiality which means that our research findings cannot be hauled into a courtroom if the insurer were to go to that length. Consequently, those of you reading this book who have already donated DNA to a research study please rest assured that, so far as we are aware, no bad consequences will happen to you as a result of this very-much-appreciated altruistic for-the-good-of-humanity endeavor. Both authors engage in research related to kidney disease and appreciate more than words can ever express the selfless kindness of our research subjects who have given their blood, urine, and DNA. Our studies address why it is that the kidney disease progresses and why there is so much else that goes awry when kidney function declines over time.

If you are considering having a genetic test done for a kidney disease, such as adult polycystic kidney disease, what do you need to do next? Our suggestion is to point your browser to www.ornl.gov/sci/techresources/Human_Genome/medicine/genetest.shtml.

From this single site, you will have virtually all of your questions answered regarding the regulations surrounding genetic testing, whether insurance covers it, the ethics involved, and the nuts and bolts associated with undergoing such testing. Genetic testing is still fairly new for most physicians, and many may not know where testing is actually done. To see if there is a lab near you that does the testing, go to www.genetests.org.

Choose "Laboratory Directory," enter the disorder and the state you live in or near. Although we are somewhat loathe to do this, there is a site you can recommend that your doctor check out which provides some very useful guidance on genetic testing in clinical medical practice. It's not limited to doctors so you're welcome to peruse it as well. Its located at http://www.genetests.org/servlet/access?id=INSERTID&key=INSERTKEY&fcn=y&filename=/tools/index.html.

If you don't want to type in this awkward 100 character website, look very carefully at the www.genetests.org website on the right hand side of the home page and you will see a link that says "Visit GENETIC TOOLS." Click that and you'll save yourself some finger strain!

Following the logic in this website choose the "Teaching Cases" tab and opt for "**Autosomal dominant**" under the heading of Indexed by Mode of Inheritance. Pick the last case, which is 33. This is a very relevant clinical example of adult polycystic kidney disease. There is lots of information at the end of the case that can help point you to further information.

Autosomal dominant

Inheritance of a genetic condition in an autosomal dominant pattern which means that each offspring has a 50% chance of inheriting the disease.

Further Information

149

Glossary

A

Acute kidney injury: Acute decline in kidney function is termed acute renal failure or acute kidney injury. Many causes of acute kidney injury are reversible.

Acute renal failure: Another term for acute kidney injury.

Acute tubular necrosis (ATN): A form of acute kidney injury or acute renal failure. ATN is the death of tubular cells, which may result when tubular cells do not get enough oxygen (ischemic ATN) or when they have been exposed to a toxic drug or molecule (nephrotoxic ATN). Fortunately, new tubular cells usually replace those that have died. The tubular cells of the kidneys undergo a continuous cycle of cell death and renewal, much like the cells of the skin.

Adrenal glands: The two small endocrine glands located just above the kidneys. The adrenal glands secrete sex hormones, cortisol, and adrenaline (epinephrine).

ADH: An antidiuretic hormone which acts in the kidney to increase the absorption of water from the kidney into the blood.

Albumin: A component of protein in the blood, low levels of serum albumin reflect poor nutritional status.

Alkalinize: To increase the alkali component or the pH in the blood or urine by adding a bicarbonate-based agent.

Amino acids: The smaller molecules that are joined to form proteins.

Angioplasty: Vascular intervention when dye is injected into an artery and, if the artery is narrowed, the vessel is opened up by inflating a ballon in the artery.

Angiotensin converting enzyme inhibitor (ACEI): A commonly used drug that blocks the renin-angiotensin system. ACE inhibitors are a type of blood pressure medication that also reduces protein in the urine in patients with chronic kidney disease. Can cause a chronic cough in some patients.

Angiotensin receptor blocker (ARB): Another commonly used drug that also blocks the renin-angiotensin system at a different receptor. ARBs are a type of blood pressure medication that also reduces protein in the urine and is commonly used in patients with diabetic kidney disease.

Antibiotics: Medications prescribed to treat infections.

Antibody: Proteins that are produced by the immune system in response to foreign substances called antigens. Each antibody is unique and defends the body against one specific type of antigen.

Arteriovenous fistula (AVF): Dialysis vascular access that is surgically created for use to receive dialysis. A native artery and vein are surgically joined together to form the arteriovenous fistula.

Arteriovenous graft: Dialysis vascular access when a synthetic piece of foreign material is used to join an artery to a vein to create a vascular access.

Arthritis: Inflammation of the joints.

Atheroemboli: Tiny pieces of cholesterol that can deposit in distant organs and cause renal failure.

Atrial septal defect: Congenital cardiac malformation of the atrium with a defect between the right and left sides of the atrium.

Autosomal dominant: Inheritance of a genetic condition in an autosomal dominant pattern that means that each offspring has a 50% chance of inheriting the disease.

B

Bariatric: Pertaining to weight.

Bicarbonate: Alkali content in the blood which is measured with a blood test.

Biopsy: A piece of tissue removed from the body and examined for abnormalities.

Bowman's space: The space surrounding the glomerulus of each nephron or kidney "fileter" unit.

C

Cadaver transplant: Organ is donated from a deceased donor or cadaver donor.

Calcineurin inhibitor: Specific type of medication that is given to suppress the immune system after receiving an organ transplant.

Calcification: Excess deposition of calcium usually in blood vessels.

Carbohydrates: A common substance in foods that are broken down in the body to simple sugars and are a major source of energy for the body.

Cardiac catheterization: Procedure where dye is injected through the groin and then travels into the arteries of the heart to assess for narrowing and deposition of cholesterol plaques in the coronary arteries.

Casts: Protein that precipitates in the urine to form protein complexes or casts.

Cardiovascular: Relating to the heart or blood vessels.

Catheter: A tube that can be inserted into a body cavity.

CellCept: A drug that suppresses the immune system and is used in treatment of certain kidney diseases such as lupus and after kidney transplant.

Centrifuge: A piece of equiptment, driven by a motor, that puts an object in rotation around a fixed axis. Urine can be placed in a centrifuge to separate substances of different densities. The urine is spun or rotated on high speed for five minutes.

Chemotherapy: A form of medication that can be given orally or through a vein for cancer therapy and for some autoimmune diseases to suppress the immune system.

Cholesterol: A form of lipid important in heart disease. Cholesterol is the basis for sex hormones and bile, but it is also a substance that can accumulate in the lining of blood vessels and cause blockages.

Cholesterol emboli: Small pieces of cholesterol that break off from a plaque and deposit in distant organs.

Chromosomes: Thread-like strands that contain hundreds, or even thousands, of genes.

Chronic kidney disease: Longstanding damage to the kidneys or chronic kidney failure.

Classes of blood pressure medications: There are about eight classes of blood pressure medicines (see Figure 4). ACE inhibitors block the angiotensin-converting enzyme, which reduces the production of angiotensin-II. Angio-tensin receptor blockers (ARBs) block the binding of angiotensin-II to its receptor (see Receptor) on the blood vessel cell. Alpha1-blockers inhibit adrenaline effects on the blood vessel. Beta-blockers inhibit adrenaline effect on heart muscles. Alpha2-agonists (like clonidine) suppress adrenergic activity. Calcium channel blockers directly relax arterial blood vessels by blocking channels through which calcium enters blood vessels cells. Vasodilators also directly relax blood vessels.

Clinical trials: This is considered the best way to demonstrate the benefits of treatment. In a clinical trial a group of people with a finding (like hypertension) are randomly assigned one or another treatment (usually without the nature of the treatment being known to the doctors conducting the study or the patients taking the treatment: this is called "blinding") and followed for a long time to see if one treatment has better outcomes (like less strokes, for example) compared with the other treatment.

Clonal: Multiple identical copies of a DNA sequence.

Complement levels: Proteins measured in the blood that are decreased in autoimmune diseases.

Conceive: When a female becomes pregnant.

Conn's Syndrome: Primary hyperaldosteronism due to overproduction of aldosterone from an adrenal tumor or adenoma.

Creatine: A compound the body synthesizes and then utilizes to store energy (see Creatinine).

Creatinine: A compound formed by the metabolism of creatine, found in muscle tissue and blood and normally excreted in the urine as a metabolic waste. Measurement of creatinine levels in the blood is used to evaluate kidney function.

Crystal: Precipitate that is seen under a microscope when looking at the urine in a patient with kidney stones.

Cyst: An abnormal membranous sac in the body containing a gaseous, liquid, or semisolid substance.

Cystinuria: Abnormal accumulation of cystine in the urine.

Cytokines: Any of several regulatory proteins, such as the interleukins and lymphokines, that are released by cells of the immune system and act as intercellular mediators in the generation of an immune response. Also called chemokine.

Cytoxan: A drug that suppresses the immune system and is used in treatment of certain kidney diseases such as lupus and in certain cancers.

D

Deceased donor transplant: Organ transplant from a deceased or cadaver donor.

Diabetes insipidus: A rare disease resulting from a deficiency of vasopressin (the pituitary hormone that regulates the kidneys) or inability receptors in the kidney to utilize vasopressin; the disease is characterized by the chronic excretion of large amounts of pale dilute urine which results in dehydration and extreme thirst.

Diabetes mellitus: A chronic disease caused by insufficient production of insulin and resulting in abnormal metabolism of carbohydrates, fats, and proteins. The disease, which typically appears in childhood or adolescence, is called type I diabetes and is characterized by increased sugar levels in the blood and urine, excessive thirst, frequent urination, acidosis, and wasting. Type I diabetes is always treated with insulin. Type II diabetes is usually diagnosed in adulthood and is associated with obesity and can be treated with insulin or oral medications to lower blood sugar levels.

Diabetic nephropathy: Chronic kidney disease due to diabetes.

Dialysis: A medical procedures to remove wastes or toxins from the blood and adjust fluid and electrolyte imbalances in patients with kidney failure or end stage renal disease.

Dialyzer: The filter that is used to filter waste products and fluid during the hemodialysis process.

Dipstick: A chemically sensitive strip of paper used to identify one or more constituents (as glucose or protein) of urine by immersion into a urine specimen.

Direct renin inhibitors: A new class of drugs that inhibit renin and are also used for the treatment of high blood pressure.

Diuretic: A substance or medication that causes an increase in urine excretion. Caffeine is an example of a naturally occurring mild diuretic. Hydrochlorothiazide, or HCTZ, is an example of a prescription diuretic.

DNA: A nucleic acid that carries the genetic information in the cell and is capable of self-replication and synthesis of RNA. DNA consists of two long chains of nucleotides, the sequence of nucleotides determines individual hereditary characteristics.

Double blind study: A clinical study in which neither the participants nor the researchers know which participants are assigned to a certain treatment group.

E

eGFR: Estimated GFR or glomerular filtration rate

Endocrine glands: Glands that secrete specific hormones, which have a specific effect on specific organs; for example, insulin is secreted by the pancreas and is responsible for metabolism of glucose.

Endocrinology: A branch of medicine that specifically deals with disorders of the endocrine system and its specific secretion of hormones.

Endothelial function: Functional ability of the lining of blood vessels.

Endothelium: A thin layer of flat epithelial cells that lines the lymph vessels, blood vessels, and the inner cavities of the heart.

Erythropoietin: A glycoprotein secreted by the kidneys that stimulates the production of red blood cells.

F

Fibromuscular Dysplasia: Abnormal proliferation of the muscular component of the artery resulting in narrowing of the renal artery lumen.

G

Gadolinium: Contrast agent or dye injected with MRI.

Gammaglobulin: A type of protein found in the blood. When gammaglobulins are extracted from the blood of many people and combined, they can be used to prevent or treat infections.

Gene: A hereditary unit consisting of a sequence of DNA that occupies a specific location on a chromosome and determines a particular characteristic in an organism. Genes undergo mutation when their DNA sequence changes.

Gestational: Having to do with pregnancy.

Glomerular filtration rate (GFR): Determines level of kidney function and stage of kidney disease.

Glomeruli: These are the tiny filter units in each kidney that initiate the formation of urine. In health they allow only the liquid part of blood to be filtered, and a barrier against protein or cells like red blood cells appearing in the urine.

Glomerulonephritis: Inflammation of the glomeruli of the kidney; characterized by decreased production of urine and by the presence of blood and protein in the urine and by edema.

Gout: A disturbance of uric-acid metabolism occurring chiefly in males, characterized by painful inflammation of the joints, especially of the feet and hands, and arthritic attacks resulting from elevated levels of uric acid in the blood and the deposition of urate crystals around the joints. The condition can become chronic and result in deformity.

Gravid: Pregnant state.

H

Hematuria: Blood in the urine.

Hemodialysis: Dialysis of the blood to remove toxic substances or metabolic wastes from the bloodstream; used in the case of kidney failure.

Hemoglobin: Iron-containing protein present in the blood that is contained in red blood cells and gives the cells the red color and also is a transporter of oxygen in the blood.

Hemoglobin A1C: Measured in the blood of diabetics to assess long-term sugar control by measuring glycosylated hemoglobin.

Hollenhorst Plaques: Cholesterol plaques seen in the retina or the back of the eyes due to deposition of atheroemboli or cholesterol emboli.

Hormones: Chemicals made by glands like the adrenal glands or the pancreas that signal other tissue to function in a particular manner. For example insulin is a hormone made by the pancreas, which, when released into the blood, stimulates the liver (and other tissues) to take up glucose (sugar) from the blood and store it. Hormones can also be made in the kidney.

Hydrocephalus: A usually congenital condition in which an abnormal accumulation of fluid in the cerebral ventricles causes enlargement of the skull and compression of the brain, destroying much of the neural tissue.

Hydronephrosis: Distention and dilation of the renal pelvis, usually caused by obstruction of the free flow of urine from the kidney.

Hyperfiltration: A condition when the kidney has increased processing of fluids through the kidney.

Hypertension: Also called high blood pressure. Hypertension is a circumstance in which a person's blood pressure has been shown to be consistently at or above 140/90 mm Hg. Hypertension is a leading risk factor for stroke, heart disease, kidney disease, and peripheral circulation problems.

I

Immunoglobulin: A protein produced by plasma cells which play an essential role in the body's immune system. These proteins attach to foreign substances like bacteria and assist in destroying them.

Inflammation: This term refers to the ability of a hormone, or a germ like a bacteria or virus, or some other influence to cause a reaction in the body that involves some aspect of the immune system. The result of this reaction is often a buildup of scar or plaque. Inflammation is thought to play a big role in hardening of the arteries.

Insulin: A hormone produced in the pancreas that regulates the amount of sugar in the blood by stimulating cells, especially liver and muscle cells, to absorb and metabolize glucose. Insulin also stimulates the conversion of blood glucose into glycogen and fat, which are the body's chief sources of stored carbohydrates.

Insulin resistance: A situation in which insulin has difficulty promoting sugar uptake into body cells (the cells are resistant). High levels of insulin and sometimes blood sugar results. People with insulin resistance are at higher risk for developing diabetes.

Interstitial nephritis: Inflammation of the kidney usually due to certain drugs such as antibiotics and sulpha-containing drugs.

Interstitium: The supporting tissue of the kidney.

Iothalamate: Substance used to measure glomerular filtration rate for more accurate assessment of kidney function.

Islet cells: Cells in the pancreas that produce insulin.

K

Kidney biopsy: A procedure usually performed with ultrasound guidance to obtain a small piece or core of kidney tissue, which is then examined under a microscope to assess the cause of a patient's kidney disease.

Kidney donation: A procedure when a person donates one of his or her kidneys to a patient with kidney failure. The donor is often a relative of the person who receives the kidney.

Kidney transplant: A procedure where a patient with severe kidney failure receives a kidney transplant either from a cadaver or deceased donor or a living donor who is often a relative or spouse.

Kidney stones: Stones that form due to aggregation of crystals in the kidney and urinary tract. Most kidney stones contain calcium.

Kidney ultrasound: The use of ultrasonic waves for diagnostic or therapeutic purposes, specifically to image the kidney and assess the size of the kidney and whether stones or obstruction is present.

L

Lactic acidosis: Abnormal accumulation of increased lactic acid levels in the blood.

Laser surgery: Surgery that is performed with a specific type of laser to treat eye disease in diabetics or diabetic retinopathy.

LDL: A lipoprotein that transports cholesterol in the blood; composed of a moderate amount of protein and a large amount of cholesterol; high levels are thought to be associated with increased risk of coronary heart disease and atherosclerosis. LDL cholesterol is also known as the "bad" cholesterol and a high level in the blood is thought to be related to various pathogenic conditions.

Lithotripsy: The procedure of crushing a stone in the urinary bladder or urethra by means of a lithotriptor, a device that passes shock waves through a water-filled tub in which the patient sits. The resulting stone fragments are small enough to be expelled in the urine.

Livedo reticularis: A purplish network-patterned discoloration of the skin caused by dilation of capillaries and venules. This can be seen in patients with atheroemboli.

Living related transplant: An organ transplant from a living donor who is related, i.e., is a sibling, parent, or child of the kidney recipient.

Lupus (SLE): A chronic generalized connective tissue disorder, ranging from mild to fulminating, marked by skin eruptions, arthralgia, arthritis, leukopenia, anemia, visceral lesions, neurologic manifestations, lymphadenopathy, fever, and other constitutional symptoms. Typically, there are many abnormal immunologic phenomena with low complement levels and presence of antinuclear antibodies.

M

Malnutrition: Poor nutritional status due to deficiencies in the diet.

Metabolism: The minimal energy expended to maintain respiration, circulation, peristalsis, muscle tonus, body temperature, glandular activity, and the other vegetative functions of the body.

Monoclonal gammopathy of undetermined significance (MGUS): Abnormal accumulation of monoclonal proteins in the blood.

Microalbuminuria: A type of albuminaria that is characterized by relatively low levels of albumin in the urine (between 30 and 300 mg in 1 day). The increase in albumin secretion is generally too small to be detected by a conventional dipstick test but can indicate the beginnings of kidney disorders, especially those related to diabetes.

mm Hg: The abbreviation for millimeters (mm) of mercury (chemical symbol is Hg), the units in which blood pressure is measured.

Multidisciplinary team: A team approach often involving a few different physicians, nurses, dietitian, social worker, and other health-care workers who all work together to come up with and implement a treatment management plan.

Myeloma: A disseminated type of plasma cell dyscrasia characterized by multiple bone marrow tumor foci and secretion of an M component, manifested by skeletal destruction, pathologic fractures, bone pain, the presence of anomalous circulating immunoglobulins, Bence Jones proteinuria, and anemia.

Myoglobin: The oxygen-transporting protein of muscle, resembling blood hemoglobin in function but with only one heme as part of the myoglobin.

N

Nephritis: Inflammation of the kidney.

Nephrogenic systemic fibrosis: Nephrogenic fibrosing dermopathy or nephrogenic systemic fibrosis is a rare and serious syndrome that involves fibrosis of skin, joints, eyes, and internal organs. Its cause is not fully understood, but it seems to be associated with exposure to gadolinium (which is frequently used as a contrast substance for MRIs) in patients with severe kidney failure. It does not have a genetic basis.

Nephrologist: A physician who is a kidney or renal specialist.

Nephron: The nephron is the functional unit of the kidney, responsible for the actual purification and filtration of the blood. There are approximately one million nephrons in each kidney.

Nephropathy: Pertaining to harmful effects on the kidney.

Neuropathy: Neuropathy is usually short for peripheral neuropathy, meaning a disease of the peripheral nerve or nerves.

NSAID: A non-steroidal anti-inflammatory drug. These drugs are used for arthritis and pain management, examples include ibuprofen, naproxen, and aspirin.

O

Occult: Not manifest or detectable by clinical methods alone and also not present in macroscopic amounts.

Oxalate: Oxalate is found in many foods and combines with calcium to form kidney stones.

P

Parathyroid glands: The parathyroid glands are small endocrine glands in the neck, usually located behind the thyroid gland, which produce parathyroid hormone. In rare cases the parathyroid glands are located within the thyroid glands. Most often there are four parathyroid glands, but some people have six or even eight.

Parathyroid hormone: A hormone which is secreted from the parathyroid gland and controls the body's metabolism of calcium and phosphorus and is involved in bone metabolism.

Patent ductus arteriosus (PDA): A congenital heart defect wherein a child's ductus arteriosus fails to close after birth. Symptoms include shortness of breath and cardiac arrhythmia, and may progress to congestive heart failure if left uncorrected.

Pathogenesis: The mechanism by which a certain factor causes disease (pathos = disease, genesis = development).

Peripheral vascular disease (PVD): Peripheral vascular disease (PVD) or peripheral artery disease (PAD) is a collator for all diseases caused by the obstruction of large peripheral arteries, which can result from atherosclerosis, inflammatory processes leading to stenosis, an embolism, or thrombus formation. It causes either acute or chronic ischemia.

Peritoneal dialysis: Peritoneal dialysis works on the principle that the peritoneal membrane that surrounds the intestine can act as a natural semipermeable membrane and that if a specially formulated dialysis fluid is instilled around the membrane then dialysis can occur, by diffusion. Excess fluid can also be removed by osmosis, by altering the concentration of in the fluid.

pH: pH is a measure of the acidity or alkalinity of a solution.

Placebo: Usually an inactive substance that contains no medication or active ingredient to be given to participants in a clinical trial to determine the effectiveness of a particular medication or substance.

Plaque: An area of hardening in the blood vessel.

Plasma cells: Plasma cells (also called plasma B cells or plasmocytes) are cells of the immune system that secrete large amounts of antibodies.

Plasmapharesis: Plasmapheresis (from the Greek plasma, something molded, and apheresis, taking away) is the removal, treatment, and return of (components of) blood plasma from blood circulation. It is thus an extracorporeal therapy. The method can also be used to collect plasma for further manufacturing into a variety of medications.

Polycystic kidney disease (PKD): (also known as polycystic kidney syndrome). A progressive, genetic disorder of the kidneys. It is characterized by the presence of multiple cysts (hence, "polycystic") in both kidneys. The disease can also damage the liver, pancreas, and, rarely, the heart and brain. The two major forms of polycystic kidney disease are distinguished by their patterns of inheritance. Autosomal dominant polycystic kidney disease (ADPKD) is generally a late-onset disorder characterized by progressive cyst development and bilaterally enlarged kidneys with multiple cysts. Kidney manifestations in this disorder include renal function abnormalities, hypertension, renal pain, and renal insufficiency.

Preeclampsia: A situation, usually arising after the 20th week of pregnancy, characterized by increased blood pressure, ankle swelling, and proteinuria (see Proteinuria) in a pregnant woman.

Prescription: An instruction from a licensed clinician like a physician, an advanced practice nurse, a midwife, or a physician's assistant that provides for a medication or device to be issued by a pharmacy.

Primary hyperaldosteronism: Autonomous secretion of the hormone aldosterone either due to a unilateral benign adrenal tumor (or adenoma) or due to bilateral adrenal hyperplasia due to overproduction of aldosterone by both adrenal glands.

Prostate: The prostate is an exocrine gland of the male mammalian reproductive system.

Protein: Proteins are large organic compounds made of amino acids arranged in a linear chain and joined together by peptide bonds. The sequence of amino acids in a protein is defined by a gene and encoded in the genetic code.

Proteinuria: The presence of protein in the urine. Protein is not usually detected in the urine of healthy individuals.

R

Receptor: This term usually refers to a protein that is anchored on the surface of a cell that specifically attracts a certain chemical or hormone. For example, the insulin receptor binds insulin from the bloodstream and once the binding

occurs, a series of reactions in the cell make possible the uptake of sugar (glucose) into that cell. The insulin receptor does not bind adrenaline, for example, so we typically say that receptors are choosy about who they are willing to partner with. Said another way we typically assert that receptors are specific in the ligands (chemicals/hormones) they bind.

Renal: Pertaining to the kidney.

Renal artery stenosis: Narrowing of one or both the renal arteries.

Renin: Renin is a circulating enzyme released mainly by juxtaglomerular cells in the juxtaglomerular apparatus of the kidneys in response to low blood volume.

Resistance: A term carried over from the world of physics. In electricity there are three forces. There is a certain amount of moving force, a certain amount of flow, and certain amount of resistance to flow that are related by this formula: Force = Flow $\times$ Resistance.

Retinopathy: Pertaining to harmful effects in the back of the eye (i.e., the retina).

S

Secondary hyperparathyroidism: Increased secretion of parathyroid hormone from the parathyroid glands due to overactivation in patients with chronic kidney disease due to vitamin D deficiency.

Statin: The statins (or HMG-CoA reductase inhibitors) form a class of hypolipidemic agents, used as pharmaceutical agents to lower cholesterol levels in people with or at risk of cardiovascular disease. They lower cholesterol by inhibiting the enzyme HMG-CoA reductase.

Stent: The main purpose of a stent is to counteract significant decreases in vessel or duct diameter by acutely propping open the conduit by a mechanical scaffold or stent. Stents are often used to alleviate diminished blood flow to organs and extremities beyond an obstruction in order to maintain an adequate delivery of oxygenated blood. Although the most common use of stents is in coronary arteries, they are widely used in other natural body conduits, such as central and peripheral arteries and veins, bile ducts, esophagus, colon, trachea or large bronchi, ureters, and urethra.

Sympathetic: This term refers to that part of the involuntary nervous system that increases heart rate and increases blood pressure.

T

Tophus: (Latin: "stone," plural tophi) is a deposit of crystallized monosodium urate in people with longstanding hyperuricemia. At this stage, most have already developed symptoms of the associated crystal arthopathy known as gout.

Tunneled dialysis catheter: A permanent catheter that is inserted usually into the internal jugular vein in order to receive dialysis. The catheter is tunneled under the skin to prevent infection.

U

Ultrasound: Renal ultrasound is a special X-ray of the kidneys that does not involve exposure to radiation. A probe with gel is placed on the patient's back and an image is projected that can give important information about your kidneys including the size of the kidneys, if any obstruction to urine flow is present, or if kidney stones are present. The ultrasound is painless.

United Network for Organ Sharing (UNOS): The United Network for Organ Sharing (UNOS) is a non-profit, scientific and educational organization that administers the nation's only Organ Procurement and Transplantation Network (OPTN), established by the U.S. Congress in 1984.

Uremia: A term used to loosely describe the illness accompanying kidney failure. In kidney failure, urea and other waste products, which are normally excreted into the urine, are retained in the blood. Early symptoms include anorexia and lethargy, and late symptoms can include decreased mental acuity and coma.

Uremic: Showing symptoms of nausea, vomiting, weight loss, decreased appetite, and fatigue associated hitw renal failure that is severe enough to consider starting dialysis. These symptoms are thought to be caused by accumulation or build up of kidney toxins.

Ureters: The ducts that carry urine from the kidneys to the urinary bladder, passing anterior to the psoas major. The ureters are muscular tubes that can propel urine along, in the adult, the ureters are usually 25–30 cm long.

Uric acid: The end product of nitrogen metabolism. High levels of uric acid in the blood are associated with increased risk of uric acid kidney stones and gout.

Urinary tract infections (UTI): An infection of the bladder.

Urine dipstick: A urine dipstick is usually made of paper or cardboard and is impregnated with reagents that indicate some feature of the liquid by changing color. For example, urine dipsticks are used to test urine samples for hemoglobin, nitrite (produced by bacteria in a urinary tract infection), glucose, and occasionally urobilinogen or ketones.

V

Vascular: Refers to blood vessels. It usually, but not always, refers to the artery type of blood vessels in particular.

Vein mapping: A procedure done with ultrasound, which defines the vessels in a patient's arms. This is done prior to making a surgical decision regarding the type of vascular access placement in a patient who is preparing for hemodialysis.

Vitamin D: A group of fat-soluble prohormones, the two major forms of which are vitamin D2 (or ergocalciferol) and vitamin D3 (or cholecalciferol). Vitamin D3 is produced in skin exposed to sunlight, specifically ultraviolet B radiation. Vitamin D plays an important role in the maintenance of organ systems. Vitamin D regulates the calcium and phosphorus levels in the blood, promotes bone formation and mineralization, inhibits parathyroid hormone secretion from the parathyroid gland, and also affects the immune system.

Index

101–102
blood count, 102–103
blood in urine, 10–11, 15–16
    kidney stones and, 128
blood pressure
    connection to kidney disease, 36–40.
        See also hypertension
    diagnosing kidney disease with,
        60–61
    guidelines for, 43–44
    having one kidney and, 3
    kidney maintenance of, 2–3
blood sugar control, 61–62
    metformin (Glucophage), 70–72
blood vessel walls, 39–40
body weight, 67, 72, 110–111
Bowman's space, 28

C

cadaver transplant. *See* deceased donor
        transplant (DDT)
calcification of blood vessels, 108
calcineurin inhibitors, defined, 72
calcium channel blockers (CCBs), 41
calcium levels, 107, 108, 113
    preventing kidney stones, 129,
        131–132
caloric intake and expenditure, 110–111
carbohydrates, 96, 110–111
cardiac catheterization, 90–91
cardiac events, chronic kidney disease
        and, 105, 125–126
casts in urine, 27–29
catheter, defined, 142
causes of kidney disease
    antibiotics, 79–80
    bladder infection, 92–93
    cardiac catheterization, 90–91
    diabetes, 60–61
    gadolinium dye, 80–82
    lupus nephritis, 86–90
    myeloma, 93–94
    NSAIDs, 78–79
    PCKD. *See* polycystic kidney disease
CCBs (calcium channel blockers), 41

centrifuge, defined, 16
cephalosporin, 79
chemotherapy for lupus treatment,
        88–89
chiropractor, 122
cholesterol, defined, 20
cholesterol emboli, 90–91
chromosomes, defined, 75
chronic kidney disease, 108–109
    defined, 33
    irreversibility of, 108–109
    NSAID use and, 78–79, 121
    risk for cardiac events, 125–126
cigarette use, 47, 67
citric acid, kidney stones and, 134
CKD. *See* chronic kidney disease
clinical trials, defined, 43
Cockcroft and Gault equation, 74–75
coffee, kidney stones and, 131
colic, 5
complement levels, defined, 88
Conn's syndrome, 54–55
consultation with dieticians, 111
consultation with specialist, when
        appropriate, 23–25
contrast with CT scans and MRIs,
        80–82
controlling blood pressure, 59–60. *See
        also* hypertension
creatinine levels, 14–15
    reduced GFR, 21–23
    when to talk to doctor, 16–17
crystals, defined, 28
CT scans, gadolinium dye for, 80–82
cystinuria, defined, 128
cysts on kidney. *See* polycystic kidney
        disease
cytokines, 66

D

darbepoetin (Aranesp), 103–104
deceased donor transplant (DDT), 123
    defined, 115
diabetes insipidus, 8
diabetes mellitus, 6, 52–54, 57–75

defined, 2
ESAs (erythropoietin stimulating
agents), 103
estimated GFR (glomerular filtration
rate), 19–21
Cockcroft and Gault equation vs.,
74–75
ethics of organ sharing, 125
exercise, 110–111

F

failure, renal, 137–144
baseline and long-term kidney
function, 140–141
family history
kidney disease, 6
kidney stones, 128
PCKD (polycystic kidney disease),
85–86
family, kidney transplants from, 124
fertility, chronic kidney diseases and, 33
fibromuscular dysplasia (FMD), 48
filtering waste product, 2
kidney function and, 17. *See also* GFR
(glomerular filtration rate)
protein in urine, 12–14
flow of urine. *See* urine
fluid intake, 7–8, 100, 110–111
hemodialysis and, 117
preventing kidney stones, 100, 129,
131
FMD (fibromuscular dysplasia), 48
focal proliferative glomerulonephritis
(FPGN), 87–88
chemotherapy needs, 89
food. *See* dietary change to treat kidney
disease
friends, kidney transplants from, 124
functions of kidneys, 2–3, 39
abnormalities in. *See* diagnosing
kidney disease
baseline function, 140–141
measuring. *See* measuring kidney
function
stages of, 19–21

G

GABA receptor, 69
gadolinium dye, 80–82
gamma globulins, defined, 92
Gatorade kidney stones and, 100, 131,
132
genetic testing, 147–149
genetics. *See* inheritance (familial)
gestational age, defined, 45
GFR (glomerular filtration rate), 17–19
estimated (eGFR), 19–21, 51–52,
74–75
production of urine and, 33–34
when to talk to specialist, 23–25
glomerular filtration rate. *See* GFR
glomeruli, defined, 17
glomerulonephritis (GN), defined, 87
chemotherapy needs, 89
glomerulus, 28
Glucophage (metformin), 70–71
gout, 133–134
grapefruit juice, kidney stones and, 131
gravid, defined, 32
gross hematuria, 15

H

HD. *See* hemodialysis
heart disease and stroke, reduced kidney
function and, 22
hematuria (blood in urine), 10–11,
15–16
kidney stones and, 128
hemodialysis (HD), 117–118. *See also*
dialysis
defined, 82, 114
performing at home, 120–121
peritoneal dialysis vs., 118
hemoglobin
defined, 16
with erythropoietin, 104–105
hemoglobin A1C, 100
HHD. *See* home hemodialysis
high blood pressure. *See* hypertension
Hollenhorst plaques, 91
home hemodialysis (HHD), 117–118,